INBORN POWERS
OF HUMAN BEINGS

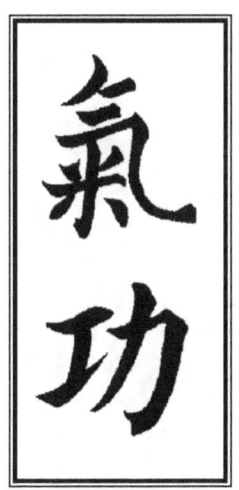

Carlos Ruiz Poleo

First English Edition
Copyright © 2014 by Carlos Ruiz Poleo
All rights reserved.

ISBN: 1495450171
ISBN: 9781495450174
Library of Congress Control Number: 2014902476
CreateSpace Independent Publishing Platform
North Charleston, South Carolina

First Spanish Edition
"Como los Humanos Manejan La Energía Sutil,
(O algo Llamado Chi-Kung)"
Centro Editor
Caracas, Septiembre 2010
Legal Dep.: If25220101502961
© Carlos Ruiz Poleo

Printed in

Dedication

To my offspring, grandchildren, relatives, and friends.

Acknowledgements

Special thanks to my Chinese friends: Master Tian Sheng Wu, Mr. Luo Liecheng, Ms. Huan Xiu Hong, Mr. Yaoming Xu, Ms. Bin Xu, and Mr. Zhuo Kai Mou.

Contents

Preface

Many anomalous phenomena happen in our lives for which science has not yet been able to provide a full and acceptable explanation. Many of these spontaneous or unexpected events that have been labeled as paranormal are actually so normal that they have been replicated in research laboratories. The world has accepted them as something that truly exists, and they are no longer considered fiction, myth, or legend. Fortunately, globalization now allows us to be aware that such events occur in many other cultures as well, and although they receive different names and their causes are attributed to various rituals or beliefs, their results or effects are the same.

Empirical knowledge is defined as knowledge that is based on or derived from observation or experiment but is not supported by proven scientific theories. But continuous practical applications of empirical knowledge allowed the advance of civilization by making use of properties and methods that produced the expected results without knowledge of their sources.

Science has identified the forces that hold the known universe in balance: strong nuclear force, weak nuclear force, electromagnetic force, and gravitational force. With the introduction and development of quantum mechanics and in search of the explanation for paranormal events, researchers have considered the existence of an additional subtle energy. This remains a highly debatable topic in the scientific community.

But this book is not intended for the scientific community; rather it is for common people who are interested in results and applications while the issue of origins, in the meantime, is further studied by specialists.

Most important for the general public is that certain actions long considered mysterious or magical are now reproducible regardless of the beliefs or rituals used to achieve them. These facts lead us to the conclusion that manipulating subtle energy is not only possible but is in fact inherent—an inborn characteristic of human beings. As members of this species, we can control that energy at will to produce effects upon physical matter by conducting certain procedures to enhance intentionality during a so-called altered state of consciousness.

CHAPTER 1

The Normal and the Extraordinary Human Capacities

Though we take normal human capacities for granted, describing them can take some time. Everything we do effortlessly and routinely is part of our normal capacities: we think, speak, and communicate in several ways, do physical and mental work, walk, run, and jump, among many other activities. Our body regularly functions as a machine, and to keep it running, we eat, breathe, take breaks, sleep, self-heal minor injuries, and combat infections. Generally speaking, our normal capacities are linked to our five senses—taste, smell, touch, sight, and hearing.

Although these capacities are normal for everyone, our levels of them differ within a certain variable range, which means that not all humans have the same vision capacity, hearing capacity, strength, artistic ability, and so on. Some of these differences, especially the physical, are accentuated with aging. These varied capacity levels establish differences among humans. For instance, in the remote past, those with better eyesight were the archers and hunters in the tribe, and as humans evolved, those with better hearing became musicians or at least good watchmen. The same is true for physical strength. Some people run faster while others are able to lift heavier weights or jump higher and so they become outstanding athletes. So those who proclaim that all humans are born equal are spreading a utopian idea, one valid only in the context of human rights. Even if all humans are exactly equal at the time they are born, immediately after birth they start differentiating due to family, culture, religion, education, nourishment, and many other influencing factors. Humans are conscious of this difference and are constantly competing to reach or surpass the capacities of other humans. Some people say that these efforts to improve capacities are the result of the process of survival of the fittest and survival of the species as well.

Whatever human tasks that are accomplished out of the range of the accepted and known capacities are hence considered extraordinary, exceptional, paranormal, or abnormal. The recent generations grew in environments influenced by movies and cartoons. As a result, they desired to become or emulate Superman and other superheroes. Of course, what differentiates those characters from the rest of us are their extraordinary capacities. The latter generation was further influenced by books, movies, and television series related to magic, like *Harry Potter*. The influence of legends like that of the wizard Merlin in previous generations is not comparable to the high impact of the modern media in recent age groups.

When we were children, all of us wished to have extraordinary powers but soon realized they were unattainable because they were just Hollywood fiction. Although sometimes the boundary between fantasy and reality is blurred, we should realize what is really possible and what is unattainable. We would do well to remember the Serenity Prayer: "Lord grant me the serenity to accept the things I cannot change, courage to change the things I can, and wisdom to know the difference between the two." Still, there are indeed some possibilities, although limited, to make use of special or extraordinary capacities or enhance those we got at birth.

Patanjali, an ancient sage from India[1] who was versed in higher Yoga[2] (raja-yoga), developed a list of extraordinary abilities or powers. In the *Yoga Sutras*[3], which he wrote or compiled, he enumerated the following *vibhutis*[4] or *siddhis*[5], which are to common people considered extraordinary or magical:

1. knowledge of the past and future (today known as premonition, forensic telepathy, post cognition, and remote viewing)
2. comprehension of the sounds (language) of all living beings (a sort of clairaudience)
3. knowledge of previous existences
4. ability to read the minds of others (telepathy)
5. invisibility (capacity of not being seen by others)
6. ability to hinder, block or prevent third parties' abilities so they cannot hear, touch, or smell our own body
7. advance knowledge of the time of one's own death
8. ability to strengthen any attitude (such as friendship)
9. super-strength (similar to that of an elephant)

---

1 Patanjali is said to be the author of the *Yoga Sutras*. There is another Patanjali who wrote on grammar (*Mahābhāṣya*). But the literary styles and contents of the *Yogasūtras* and the *Mahābhāṣya* are entirely different, and it is been proved that they were not authored by the same person.

2 The Yoga tradition is very old. References in the *Mahābhārata*, and the *Gitā* identify three kinds of yoga. According to the late *Yogatattva Upanishad*, yoga is divided into four forms—mantra-yoga, laya-yoga, hatha-yoga, and raja-yoga—the last of which is the highest (or royal) practice.

3 The *Yoga Sūtras* of Patañjali are 196 Indian sūtras (short aphorisms) that constitute the foundational text of Yoga. Although the *Yoga Sutras* have become the most important text of Yoga, the opinion of many scholars is that Patañjali was not the creator of Yoga, which existed well before him, but merely a great expounder. In contrast to the focus on the mind in the yoga sutras, later traditions of Yoga such as hatha yoga focus on more complex *asanas*, or body postures.

4 Vibhuti may refer to glorious attributes of the divine, and in this context is translated as "all pervading," "superhuman power," "wealth," and so on.

5 Siddhis are spiritual, magical, paranormal, or supernatural powers acquired through a *sadhana* (spiritual practices), such as meditation and yoga. People whom have attained siddhis are formally known as Siddhas.

10. knowledge of hidden, remote, or subtle things (also known as psychometrics, dowsing, or clairvoyance).
11. knowledge of other worlds, spaces, or universes
12. astronomical knowledge (the location and movement of stars and planets)
13. knowledge of our body's organic systems
14. liberation from the sensations of hunger and thirst
15. vision of perfected beings (*siddhas*)
16. knowledge of all things
17. knowledge of pure consciousness (*purusha*)
18. ability to listen, touch, see, taste, and smell mentally (without physical contact)
19. ability to control the bodies of others
20. ability to float or walk on water, swamps, or similar places
21. ability to radiate a glow (aura) around the body
22. ability to hear at great distances
23. ability to master the elements (earth, water, fire, air)
24. ability to make one's body atomically small, indestructible
25. possession of a perfect view of the body in beauty, strength, grace, and brilliance
26. mastery of the senses
27. quick thinking and perception through the senses
28. supremacy over all states of existence, or omnipotence
29. superior knowledge
30. absolute freedom (*kaivalyam*)

Though some consider the items on the preceding list to be just a recount of fantasies and myths, research in the field of parapsychology and other branches of science has demonstrated the existence of many of those powers, though they may not be highly developed. We cannot cover the sun with a finger, and all of us should acknowledge that at some time in our lives, we have had experiences that cannot be explained in normal terms. At the very least, we may have read or watched reports on events beyond normal boundaries.

The term *paranormal* has been mostly used to refer to unusual psychic or mental activity. But let's look at some other so-called extraordinary actions or events, literally "beyond the ordinary." We will be dealing with the following areas of knowledge, in which extraordinary or paranormal actions have been reported:

1. Biology and health. In these fields we can observe extraordinary longevity and miraculous healings.
2. Anatomy and physiology. In the study of the human body, enhanced force (super-force) and strength far above our known capacities (super-strength) have been reported.
3. Here we observe mental and/or psychic activity or the capacity to intertwine with other humans, animals, plants, and material objects without physical contact.

Recent studies demonstrate that in general people's attitude toward paranormal phenomena has changed dramatically in the last two decades. Debate is now centered not on the existence of those paranormal capacities (which have been proved and are quite accepted) but on their causes and origins.

For comprehension of extraordinary or paranormal events, especially in the psychic field, we need to be aware of the difference between *perception* and *sensation*. The sensation we get after touching a cold object with the hands originates from a mechanism of perception through our specialized temperature-sensitive skin cells[6] that send a signal to the brain, where perception becomes a feeling of cold or heat. Sensory receptors are specialized cells in the uptake of stimuli that represent gateway information in the nervous system of an organism. Perceptions are a result of stimuli perceived in the material world by specialized receptors, so they are considered objective and realistic, but sensations or feelings,

---

6 Krause corpuscles perceive cold, and Rufino corpuscles perceive heat.

which are the product of a brain process, are deemed subjective and unrealistic. Our reactions are based on both perception and sensation, the first being quite automatic and the second more mentally conditioned.

Approaching the edge of a cliff or a balcony's railing in a tall building, we perceive the staggering height and become afraid, but in a dream we can feel the same sensation and even get the impression that we will fall into the void. The first case is a real situation while the second is an illusion that exists only in our mind. That's why we use two different verbs, *perceive* (realize) and *feel* (sense). Although feelings are subjective they are a result of brain processes and modern studies of brain function have allowed scientists to physically locate feeling centers based on the intensified activity of neurons in certain areas observed with magnetic resonance imaging (MRI) or positron-emission tomography (PET scans).

Receptors and their attached sensory system constitute what is traditionally defined as the five senses. These receivers are basically in contact with energy vibration and external environmental objects. Light, for example, is an electromagnetic vibration that is part of a larger spectrum that includes radio waves and radar, but our eyes (photoreceptors) are set up to capture only that part of the spectrum we call light and then convert it into neural impulses that are processed in the brain. Other animals, such as bats, are equipped to capture a range of different frequencies, so their mental image is not the same as ours. Even animals quite close to man—like cats and dogs—can see a different spectrum, one that includes infrared light that is invisible to us.

Some people reason that the vision of dogs, cats, tigers, and the like can be considered paranormal because these animals see at night what to us is invisible or nonexistent. This interpretation of visual perceptions can be extended to other human senses, such as smell and taste, because many animals possess the extraordinary capacity to smell and sense things that are alien or nonexistent to us. Many insects, for instance, have the ability to smell the pheromones[7] of their potential mate from miles away. You can say the same about sounds: whales and elephants communicate across many miles with ultralow sounds that we do not perceive. All this is, in a sense, extraordinary or paranormal when compared to the capacities of human beings.

The list of five senses, as traditionally defined by science, has now been extended to include about twenty. Among the twenty we find the spatial sense (the perception of our surroundings), the sense of equilibrium or balance (which allows us not fall to the ground), the sense of belonging, and many others, among which some even include the sense of humor.

Perceptions received through senses other than the established twenty are called extrasensory perceptions, or ESP. In addition to this, we have to take into consideration events related to human health, such as reports of miraculous cures or unexplainable healing. These events are frequently used by organized religions to attract followers. Catholics constantly sanctify new persons based on their supposed capacity to perform miracles, especially healing incurable patients. Thousands of people engage in pilgrimages to holy places every year to witness or receive such miracles. But Catholics do not have the exclusive rights to performing miracles. Other religions report them as well, and even primitive healers like shamans were able to perform them. While the rituals, ceremonies, and beliefs of these various groups differ, the results seem to be quite similar.

Phenomena related to super-strength and the capacity to withstand attacks that otherwise would kill or seriously damage a person have been reported by Hindu Yogis and Chinese who practice martial arts. These phenomena and the capacity to live longer and better are all the result of the same manipulation of subtle energies, which occurs when

---

7 A pheromone is a secreted or excreted chemical factor that triggers a social response in members of the same species. Pheromones are chemicals capable of acting outside the body of the secreting individual to impact the behavior of the receiving individual. There are alarm pheromones, food-trail pheromones, sex pheromones, and many others that affect behavior or physiology.

people access an altered state of consciousness (ASC) and enhance their intentionality.

In addition to our own incomprehensible physical or mental experiences, most of us have also read or heard reports of similar experiences from people we know or strangers. The occurrence of these phenomena is widespread across cultures. Doubtless existence of these experiences is recorded in many languages and cultures, and they have been mentioned in different religious manuscripts. Some, with time, have even been transformed into legends and myths.

All humans seem to have inborn capacities to accomplish such unusual actions. Inherited capacities and training make such possible, with different levels of results.

CHAPTER 2

What Has to Be Controlled?

It stands to reason that something within human control must exist that allows us to attain results and perform actions beyond those largely considered normal. That "something" seems to be a subtle form of energy that is able to act upon matter or other types of energy to change their properties and performance. So the animal to be tamed is called *subtle energy*.

Like the moon, which has many different names depending on people's languages or dialects, the subtle energy that people empirically use to accomplish abnormal actions goes by many different names as well.

In primitive tribes there was always a sorcerer-healer, one with knowledge of herbs as well as the ability to handle a hidden and mysterious force (energy) during certain rituals, both of which allowed him or her to perform unexpected healings. The fact that sorcerers or shamans did not know anything about the origin of that mysterious force did not prevent them from using it to their advantage. Still, their primitive level of knowledge meant they were unable to investigate it further, and so they focused on only the resulting effects. And since they considered it an advantageous practice, they logically thought it desirable to transmit that practical knowledge through their rituals to the next generations.

The knowledge that these warlocks had about healing herbs gave rise to our modern pharmaceutical science, and their initial control and handling of subtle energies, known to Chinese as *qi* (气)' or to Japanese as *ki*, (氣)[8] set a precedent for future generations. The Yogis in India knew that energy as *prana*. Ancient Egyptians believed that humans possessed a *ka*, or life-force, that left the body at the point of death (soul energy). Each person also had a *ba*, a set of unique spiritual characteristics. In Christian terms this invisible and incomprehensible energy was referred to in many cases as divine force or divine energy. Nowadays both Christians and Satanic sects attribute the marvels obtained by controlling this energy to either God or the devil; likewise, ancient cults or religious groups attributed so-called miracles to their in-fashion god or goddess.

In 1942, German researcher William Reich described a type of energy with all the same features, which he called *orgone*. In esoteric texts (*Isis, The Truth Revealed*) this energy is called *folhat*. Hassidic mystics refer to it as a sort of emanation or *Sephirah*, and it is also known in other cultures as élan vital, animal magnetism, OD, mana, prima materia, spiritus mundi, niter, kundalini, and more.

The pre-Socratic Greek philosopher Anaximander (6th century BC) described the existence of an energy different from the air we breathe that permeated all that exists and named it Apeiron. Diogenes of Apollonia (425 BC) then insisted that all living things shared a common energy and referred to this as *pneuma* a word whose meaning refers not only to air but also to the thinking part of the mind or spirit. Individual vital energy was described also as *thymos* and collectively as *psyche*. Democrites and his master Leucippus (one of the earliest authors of atomism theory) described the characteristics of what they called "psyche energy." Then Damascius and the neo-Platonic Simplicius established the difference between psyche and pneuma. Lastly Hippocrates referred to the energy as *enormon*, the force that provided vital energy.

---

8 Japanese use the same traditional Chinese symbol (Kanji) for this concept.

All animals, including humans, are activated by a vital energy. We must remember that our life in fact begins with the union of the vital energy transferred from our parents at the moment of fertilization, when both provide living cells (eggs and sperm) with a vital energy that lasts a limited time[9]. These living cells are thus energized but also equipped with specialized instructions to develop a specific structure, the DNA genetic code, instructions that seem to be complemented by the existence of a morphic resonance field[10].

Similarly, plants in the vegetable kingdom also provide vital energy for reproduction and survival of the species through their seeds. Like animals, they have a specific building program (DNA), and the duration of their vital energy is also limited. However, in plants this energy lasts far longer because of its ability to remain in a latent state in adverse environmental conditions. Germination will occur only when conditions become favorable to the development of life, sometimes after months or several years. Humans have introduced in vitro fertilization and sperm banks, which are in a sense comparable to these latent capacities of plant seeds.

---

9 The ejaculation inside the vagina accounts for 2 to 3 milliliters of sperm that contains between 150 and 300 million spermatozoids. The life of these is 48 to 72 hours, or an average of 60 hours. The female eggs have an average life of 36 hours.

10 Morphic resonance field is a term introduced by Rupert Sheldrake and is something all living species seem to have. It connects individuals with their kind and with "instructions" located outside our space-time dimension.

Researchers from various universities and research institutions around the world[11] today devote a great deal of financial and human resources to the investigation of the anomalous behavior of the actions of mind over matter. In the scientific community, this energy is also referred to as mind energy, subtle energy, psychic energy, anomalous energy, vital energy, life-force, *lebenskraft*, and many other names, all of which are simply different terms for the same concept.

This vital energy at a macro level is what the Hindus call *para-atman*. At a micro level it is the *atman/prana* or *cit*, an energy unit of a larger system. Historically, the *Huangdi Neijing (The Yellow Emperor's Classic of Medicine)*, written circa the second century BCE, is credited with first establishing the pathways through which the subtle energy qi (气) circulates in the human body.

For other types of energies, scientists have already established units and measurement methods like the joule (J), electron volts (eV), kilowatt-hours (kW), and Calories (C) etc. But in general the concept of vital or subtle energy is very difficult to discuss in a scientific paradigm because so far there is not a tool to measure it; and its measurement unit is not yet defined.

---

11 It is nearly impossible to include in a footnote all institutions devoted to this type of research, but I will mention the most prominent, such as the Centre for Psychophysical Studies (Nantmel, Wales, UK), the Consciousness Group of the Scientific and Medical Network, (Hartford Drive, Bristol, UK), the School of Public Health at the University of Illinois (Chicago), the Fund of Parapsychology Leonid Vasiliev (Moscow, Russia), the Princeton Engineering Anomalies Research Laboratory at Princeton University (New Jersey), the Department of Physics, University of Cambridge (Cambridge, UK), the Center for the Investigation of Consciousness (Lexington, Kentucky), the Harvard University Medical School and Human Brain Research Laboratory (Fairfield, Iowa), the Consciousness Research Laboratory, Harry Reid Center University of Nevada (Las Vegas), the Department of Psychology-Uris Hall, Cornell University (Ithaca, New York), the Cognitive Sciences Laboratory, Science Application International Corp. (Palo Alto, California), the Parapsychology Laboratory, University of Amsterdam (Holland), The Retro psychokinetic Project from University of Kent (Canterbury, UK), Rhine Research Center at Duke University (Durham, North Carolina), and The Farsight Institute, just to mention western hemisphere institutions. Including those in China, Japan, Korea, Taiwan and India would be an endless task.

To accept a new immaterial concept is something very personal and is tied to our social milieu and rooted beliefs. It is good to remember Nicolaus Copernicus (1473–1543) and Galileo Galilei (1564–1634), who were both attacked and victimized for not accepting a dogma and trying to scientifically explain that the Earth revolved around the sun, and not the other way around. They were faced with the problem of having to explain something that was against the already accepted logic: seeing the sun rise in the east and—after making its path across the sky—set in the west, people believed that the Earth was the center of the universe. Convincing people that the Earth was not flat was similarly difficult; this went against all their observations of the surrounding land and seas.

Denial is commonly used as a defense mechanism. Sigmund Freud used the term to describe the response that occurs when people are faced with a fact that is too uncomfortable to accept: they reject the fact, insisting it is not true despite sometimes overwhelming evidence. Others refer to this as dissonance or cognitive dissonance,[12] which is aroused when people are confronted with information that is inconsistent with their beliefs and so reject it.

I, like many of you, am reluctant to easily and radically exchange an existing mental framework for a new one, and I prefer to maintain a balanced opinion by asking many questions. But sometimes it seems that I surpass my own skepticism and remain reluctant to accept explanations until I am convinced that there is a true and verifiable cause. When we are faced with an idea that makes us uncomfortable or seems inconsistent, it is important to remember that we, Westerners, do not have the monopoly on truth; teachings of other cultures are also part of the heritage of humankind. Thus it is best to take the best of each culture, discarding dogmas and keeping an open mind. Doing so

---

12 Cognitive dissonance is a mental conflict that occurs when beliefs or assumptions are contradicted by new information. The concept was introduced by the psychologist Leon Festinger (1919–89) in the late fifties. He and later other researchers showed that when confronted with challenging new information, most people seek to preserve their current understanding of the world by rejecting, explaining away, or avoiding the new information or by convincing themselves that no conflict really exists. Cognitive dissonance is nonetheless considered an explanation for attitude change.

allows us to assimilate what we initially found strange and avoid what psychologists call preconditioning, or biased perception.

Dr. Dean Radin in his book *The Conscious Universe*[13] refers to the attitude of scientists when presented with new phenomena that go against established principles. He claims that in the sciences, the acceptance of new ideas follows a predictable pattern of four stages:

> ... *"In the first stage* scientists openly proclaim that the proposed idea or hypothesis is *'impossible'* because it violates the laws of science. This first stage can last from a few years to centuries, depending on to what extent it challenges the conventional established principles. *In the second stage* the skeptics timidly accept that it *'might be possible'* but that it is not very interesting and the alleged effects are very weakly supported.
>
> *In the third stage*, the mainstream realizes that not only the idea *'is possible'*, but also that its effects are much stronger and more widespread than previously imagined. *The fourth stage* is achieved when the same critics who preached dismissively their disinterest, then hypocritically proclaim that they were the first who thought of it. Ultimately no one will remember that the idea was once considered as a dangerous heresy" ...

Taking into consideration this process, we should adopt a methodology for understanding energy control by taking something from each of the sciences related to energy to be used as scaffolding in our exploration of everything related to the gathering, identification, differentiation, accumulation, control, and emission of this energy. Subsequent chapters will often refer to the "new physics" and the "new

---

13 Radin, Dean. *The Conscious Universe.* Harper Collins, 1997. I also recommend his other book, *Entangled Minds: Extrasensory Experiences in a Quantum Reality* (Paraview Pocket Books, 2006).

biology," and it is worth mentioning that the study of subtle energy requires basic knowledge in the fields of chemistry, physics, biology, cybernetics, and other areas of human knowledge, much of which we were exposed to in high school or our early college years. I advise the reader to further investigate some topics as this book could not deal in deep with every subject. Nevertheless, as mentioned before, this work is intended for the average reader and not for the scientific community so I will try to make the references as simple as possible in order to avoid any confusion or misunderstanding.

Because subtle energy can be used and controlled, people should have access to it or at least be aware of its existence, regardless of their scientific expertise. Some use this energy intuitively; others require more effort and training, and this distinction bring up an important point. There is a great difference between a *gift* (for many a *divine gift*) and a *capacity* or *ability*, although often these words are erroneously used interchangeably.

When we refer to a gift or talent, we mean something that is inborn, henceforth given to us free and benevolently and without demanding anything in return. Thus we use the term *gifted* to describe people who from their early childhood have the potential to become great musicians, composers, and performers. Others may have the gift of wisdom, fortitude, piety, creativity, and so on. The extrasensory capacities that some individuals normally and innately manifest may also be considered gifts.

On the contrary, capacities or abilities are not received, but earned or developed. They are usually the result of effort. We see this in athletes who prepare and exercise extensively to have the capacity to achieve certain skill levels (such as lifting heavy loads, jumping great distances, or winning difficult tournaments). This is also noticeable in the performing arts, music, and painting or sculpture, in which results depend on previous learning and extensive practice. Everyone would like to have the power to lift heavy weights, conduct a symphony orchestra, or be the star quarterback of a football team, but these require preparation, effort, perseverance, and commitment.

When comparing talents and abilities, we must recognize that a portion of the potential capacity could be obtained without effort. A person might be born with that potential, but in order to achieve full capacity, the remainder must be enhanced and cultivated to facilitate achievement. For example, someone who was fortunate enough to be born into a rich family will surely have economic support for whatever he or she would initiate; the person will have advantages that others haven't. If the person knows how to profit from that privilege and does not waste it, then it will be easier for him or her to achieve objectives faster or more comfortably. Of course, many do not appreciate their given advantages and miss opportunities that many others would like to have. But we must not forget that although some people could have an easier way to achieve their goals, they will never become really successful without putting forth some effort.

A quote from Louis Pasteur (1822–1895)[14] will remind us of that reality: "*Let me tell you the secret that has led me to my success…My strength lies solely in my tenacity!*"

Having in mind that we should combine our inborn talents with a continuous effort to have a better life, our following step is to define how this activity should be carried on and what the substance we would be working with is.

In order to make things easier, we will use from now on the Chinese term *qi* (气)[15] (pronounced "chi") when referring to subtle energy, a term free of religious connotations.

---

14 Pasteur is a French multifaceted scientific genius: author of germ theory, founder of vaccination, microbiology, and pasteurization, inventor of rabies vaccine.

15 Traditional Chinese 氣; Simplified Chinese 气. The Chinese written language is based on pictographs or ideographs, so to transliterate Chinese spoken sounds that could be understood or reproduced, Westerners adopted a system of European languages letters known as pinyin. In this system our sound *ch* (like in chip, cheap, and chat) is written with the letter Q.

Qi is a fundamental concept in Chinese philosophy, where it is considered the only elemental substance in the universe that possesses strength and energy. Chinese philosophy states that in the primitive stage of the formation of the known universe, there was absolutely nothing but qi. This is similar to the concept of apeiron of the ancient Greek philosophers. It is said that due to the characteristics and movement of qi, nature began to structure, and the universe was developed. Would that ancient theory have something to do with the modern theory of the big bang? The latter assumes that interstellar matter was generated from a void in which there existed only energy as the result of a tremendous shock wave. Could that primeval qi theory have something to do with the biblical texts that state that in the beginning there was nothing, and all started with a vibration (wrongly translated as "word" or "utterance")? Does it have something to do as well with the knowledge transmitted in the Egyptian book *The Kybalion*, which also tells us that in the beginning there was only vibrating energy? Could this theory of qi be associated with the modern theory of superstrings, which is based as well on vibration?

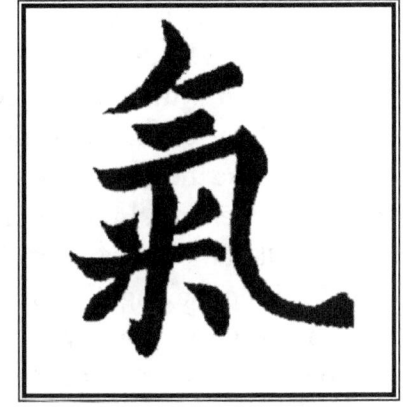

Among the words used by the Chinese to refer to the universal energy (qi) and the one used by ancient Indian sages, or rishis, for the same concept (prana) there is a remarkable similarity in properties and applications. Swami Sivananda says that prana is the total sum of all the energy contained in the universe, and in his description, its characteristics seem to match those of qi.

As mentioned before, defining intangible or invisible things is very difficult. Some people try to define qi as a form of electric energy, others consider it a magnetic type, and some believe it to be thermal energy or even a biofield. Most explanations are made by comparing it with something already known. Literally *qi* means "breath" or "vapor".

It bears a resemblance to the origin of the Sanskrit word *atman*, from which we derive our concept of soul, a word that is also similar to the Hebrew *ruach*, which translated also means "breath". In Taoism[16] qi it is considered one of the fundamental substances of the cosmos.

In Chinese the word *qi* has a more general meaning than the Western equivalent of *energy*. In traditional Chinese medicine, it is believed that life is the result of the presence of qi, and therefore they say, "To live is to have qi; dying is not having it." This word is also used in combination to define many other types of energy (electricity, magnetism, heat, or light). Thus we see how China's electric power is called *diann qi* (electric qi), and heat is called *rheh qi* (heat qi). The word *qi* is also used to express the energy state of something, especially a living being. The climate is called *tian qi* (heaven qi) because it indicates the energy state of the sky. When a person is alive, the energy of the body is called *rhen qi* (human qi). When a thing is alive, is said to have *hwo chi* (vital qi), and when it is dead, it has *syy qi* (death qi) or *goe qi* (ghost qi). Thus following the ideographic Chinese writing, the symbol for *qi* combined with others not only represents energy itself but also defines the energy's form or type.

This demonstrates that already in ancient times the Chinese were aware that energy exists in different forms and that these forms could be transformed into one another, which is essentially the principle of conservation of energy. They recognized as well that humans transfer energy to their offspring at the time of conception. This energy they called *yuan qi* (original or ancestral qi), and they called the qi acquired after birth *zong qi* (gathering qi). They also knew that eating and breathing provided us energy, called *gu qi*.

Since ancient times, the Chinese have cultivated an art or science known as Qigong [Simplified Chinese: 气功; traditional Chinese: 氣功] that enables individuals to control that specific energy. They apply this knowledge to improve life quality and longevity, to physically strengthen

---

16 Taoism, also known as Daoism, is an indigenous Chinese religion often associated with the Dao de jing (Tao Te Ching), a philosophical and political text purportedly written by Laozi (Lao Tzu) sometime in the 3rd or 4th centuries B.C.E.

the body for martial arts, to conduct healing processes, and to develop psychic capacities and powers.

So now we know more about the nonmaterial element to be controlled, but to fully understand the process, we should make a short review of three concepts: systems, energy, and vibration.

CHAPTER 3

A Review of Systems

Multiple languages that humans use to communicate orally and in writing are the result of a tacit agreement for transmitting information by using coded sounds or written symbols. The person who does not have access to those codes does not have access to information. We could experience this when we hear other people talking in a foreign language. We do not understand them because we do not know the sound or writing codes used to represent an object or action.

These agreed-upon codes, in the form of written symbols or spoken words to refer to specific objects or actions, require that partners have similar experiences related to those concepts. It is very difficult for anyone to recall an image of a thing that was never seen. I once had the opportunity to visit an Indian tribe in a remote part of the Amazon jungle. To get there—a town that was at the edge of a river—we made a long journey combining different modes of transportation, from airplanes to canoes. One of the natives, when told about our trip, understood perfectly the last part—a hike from the river to the village and the previous navigation in canoes. But what he could never understand, and what I was unable to clarify, was that part of the trip we'd made in a small airplane.

In our own cultural environments, when one refers to the moon or to any animal—a bull, for instance—problems with comprehension do not occur because the referents are familiar. Speaking about the moon worldwide is also possible, though probably with a different name, because people anywhere on the planet can see it. We could easily learn what it is called in another language if told. But a bull, something familiar to us, would be an alien concept to an isolated Eskimo or a desert dweller, as these populations do not have an image of such in their minds. We should therefore make a comparison with something they know (like a bear for the Eskimos and a camel for the desert nomad) and then establish differences by using descriptive modifiers such as adjectives or adverbs. In this way one can modify the mental image of something already registered in the brain in order to visualize the unfamiliar thing. So far this is a fairly simple task, for we have been talking about objects with preconceived or similar images and minor variations.

But this process becomes more complicated when we attempt to describe something that is understood as something different by the listener due to perceptions or biasing, what our ancestors meant when they said, "All depends on the eye of the beholder," or, in Spanish, "All depends on the color of the eyeglasses."

The preceding comments are meant to emphasize our need to speak a common language in order to avoid misunderstandings like those that occur with double-meaning jokes. The three basic concepts required to fully understand the discussion in this book are systems, energy, and vibration. Let's clarify the first.

Systems are defined using several fundamental ideas. First, all phenomena can be viewed as a web of relationships among elements. Second, all systems, whether electrical, biological, or social, have common patterns, behaviors, and properties that can be understood and used to develop greater insight into the behavior of complex phenomena.

A specialized area of knowledge to study systems behavior has been named systems theory. This helps us to determine the scope of a system by defining its boundary; this refers to choosing which entities are inside the system and which are outside (in the surrounding environment).

So, precisely defined, a system is a set of interacting or interdependent components forming an integrated whole or a set of elements (often called components) and their relationships. Three elements are present in any system: a system has *structure* (i.e., it contains parts or components that are directly or indirectly related to one another); it has *behavior*, which includes processes that transform input into output (material, energy, or data); and it has *interconnectivity* (the parts and processes are connected by structural and/or behavioral relationships). And finally a system's structure and behavior may be decomposed via subsystems[17] and sub processes to elementary parts and process steps.

In everyday conversation we use terms like *the solar system*, which comprises the sun, planets, satellites, asteroids, and some other elements; *the circulatory system*, which includes our heart, arteries, veins, and so on; and *the digestive system*, formed by our intake organs (mouth, teeth, and tongue) plus the stomach, intestines, and associated secreting glands (lever, pancreas, and more). Terms like *ecosystem* refer to many other systems, in this case subsystems constituted by animals, plants, and minerals and their interactions. Common to all systems is that their components are varied and different from one another, but all are associated in a whole. Today everything seems to belong to a system. Even *social system* is a central term in sociological systems theory.

The human body is defined by many scientists as a bio energetic system that gets its energy (qi) from food and air, and then electrochemical processes transform that energy into activities such as movement and mental actions. This bio energetic system is also affected by natural external radiations (e.g., the electromagnetic field of the earth and electric fields in the atmosphere) and artificial, human-produced radiations (e.g., magnetic fields generated by high-voltage power distribution cables, equipment radiation of X-rays and gamma rays, and radiation from microwaves, whose influence on the human body was recently discovered).

It is very important to understand very clearly the concept of *system*, as we will be dealing with our biological energetic system and the way it can interact with other external energetic systems or subsystems. I will also discuss in subsequent chapters that our "human system" is composed

---

17   A subsystem is a set of elements that is a system itself and a component of a larger system.

of three main subsystems. First is the body (the material component), which has complex subsystems forming part of it. Secondly we have the energy component. This receives many names, depending on the observer, but we will call it "the soul"; it is responsible for keeping us alive. The third subsystem controls the other two subsystems. We will call it "the spirit," though for many it's known as "higher consciousness," "higher self," or "the mind."

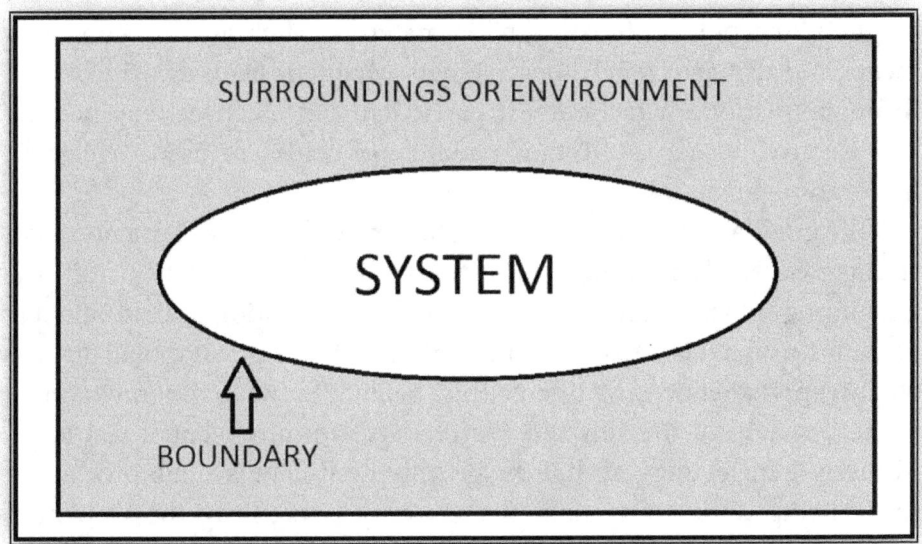

As we will be talking about systems interacting with other systems, it is worth taking a moment to clarify another term: *field*. Our interest in fields (not the green ones with cattle pasturing) is based on the evidence that a field is a complex of forces that serve as causative agents in human behavior. But what are fields?

The meaning of *field* that interests us is the one assumed by physics. All of us have heard talk about a gravitational field or a magnetic field. This could be simply imagined as a physical area or space around matter that is subject to the influence of another matter or force (energy). It has physical reality, it occupies space, it contains energy, and its presence eliminates a true vacuum. The field creates a condition in space such that when we put a particle in it, the particle "feels" a force. A field may be thought of as extending throughout the whole of space. In practice, the strength of every known field has been found to diminish with distance to the point of being undetectable. A field theory is a physical theory that describes how one or more physical fields interact with matter.

Let's take, for instance, the Earth, which produces its own magnetic field that is important in navigation. In everyday life, magnetic fields are most often encountered as invisible forces created by permanent magnets that pull on ferromagnetic materials, such as iron, cobalt, or nickel, and attract or repel other magnets. Magnetic fields are widely used throughout modern technology, particularly in electrical engineering and electro mechanics. Rotating magnetic fields are used in electric motors and generators.

The gravitational field, according to Newton's theory of gravity, has a strength inversely proportional to the square of the distance from the gravitating object. Therefore the Earth's gravitational field quickly becomes undetectable on cosmic scales. But the gravitational field is what keeps planets in orbit by creating a balance between the gravitational attraction field of the sun and the planets' spinning centrifugal force. Modern theories suggest that the gravitational field is a sub product of the existing dark matter and dark energy (which, by the way, have nothing to do with evil things) that account for more than 80 percent of the existing matter in the universe. But little else is known about this dark energy and its distribution in the solar system. Investigators recently detected a halo of dark matter around earth's equator.

A third type of field, the electric field, is linked to electrical charges by the effects on another charge. Historically, the first time that fields were taken seriously was with Faraday's lines of force [18] when describing

---

18 The concept of lines of force was introduced into physics in the 1830s by the English scientist Michael Faraday, who considered magnetic and electric effects in the region around a magnet or electric charge as a property of the region rather than an effect taking place at a distance from a cause. In physics, lines of force are the path followed by an electric charge free to move in an electric field or a mass free to move in a gravitational field, or generally any appropriate test particle in a given force field.

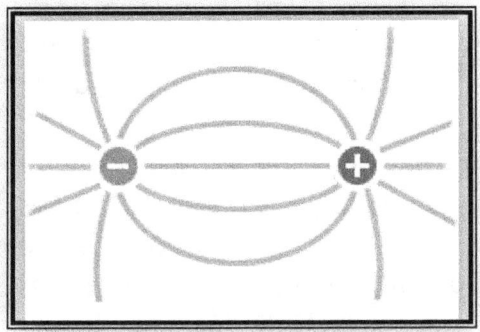

the electric field. The gravitational field was then similarly described. The electrical field force acts between two charges in the same way that the gravitational field force acts between two masses. An electric field (E) is a little bit different from a gravitational field (g). Gravitational force depends on mass whereas electrical force does not. Instead, electric force depends on charges on both objects.

A charge in empty space experiences no electric forces, but a charge placed near another charge does. The reason for this difference is that a charge creates an electric field that permeates the surrounding space and affects other nearby charges. As long as no other charge is present, an electric field does nothing. But when another charge is introduced into the field, the field exerts a force on it. The presence of an electric field can be detected by its effect on a charged object introduced into the region.

The combination of magnetic fields with electric fields creates the aptly named electromagnetic fields which actually exist beyond any doubt as demonstrated by laboratory experiments, making the field concept a supporting paradigm of modern physics. The fact that the electromagnetic field can possess momentum and energy makes it something very real. Waves of electric and magnetic energy moving together, or radiating, through space form the electromagnetic fields, invisible lines of force that surround any electrical device that is plugged in and turned on. Electric fields are produced by electric charges whereas magnetic fields are produced by the flow of current through wires or electrical devices. Electromagnetic fields are commonly associated with power lines. A person standing directly under a high-voltage transmission line may feel a mild shock when touching something that conducts electricity. These sensations are caused by the strong electric fields from the high-voltage electricity in the lines. They occur only at close range because the electric fields rapidly become weaker as the distance from the line increases. From the preceding concepts, we should be aware that our physical body and our system's energetic component (soul) are subject to proven invisible external influences.

Many experiments demonstrate the influence of magnetic fields in the migration patterns of many animal species, especially birds. These fields also influence behavior of insects. But more recent essays demonstrate that animals closer to humans (domestic animals like dogs, cats, and birds) besides smelling and hearing far better than their human companions can sense Earth's magnetic field, too. This influence on animals is the subject of study called the *magnetoreception sense*, which may help scientists better understand how that strange sense manifests in mammals. In the past we considered the practice of Eastern religions to pray or meditate while oriented to north or south to be superstition, but nowadays it would be worth studying the effect of such orientation. I myself have noticed certain differences while meditating in one place or another, and now I realize that this could be the result of my orientation.

Summarizing, the importance of systems theory and fields is that our bodies are subject to many surrounding invisible influences that cannot be ignored. Physicists are used to deal with those invisible concepts, while most of us are not. Someone told me that physicists were more prone to believe in ghosts than medical personnel due to the former being acquainted with invisible forces.

CHAPTER 4

A Review of Energy

The objective of this book is to show how humans are able to manipulate and control subtle energy for different purposes that are considered paranormal or exceptional. Such energy is known by different names, but as we will be dealing with a certain form of energy, we must clarify what that concept really means.

Difficulty arises when one tries to transmit information related to intangible or invisible things, especially when the parties involved have no common background. This is a recurring problem in all fields in which people deal with nonmaterial concepts. One such concept is energy; even physicists have not yet agreed upon a universally accepted definition for it. Compounding this problem is the fact that words have connotations or meanings in addition to their scientific senses. In many cases the original meaning is distorted for convenience—as seen in pseudoscience[19]—and this contributes to more confusion and misinterpretations.

Because of these confusion surrounding the word *energy*, it is necessary, almost imperative, that we agree on what we will be talking

---

19 Pseudoscience is a claim, belief, or practice that is presented as scientific but does not adhere to a valid scientific method, lacks supporting evidence or plausibility, cannot be reliably tested, or otherwise lacks scientific status. It is often characterized by the use of vague, contradictory, or exaggerated claims by using scientific terms out of context or by attributing them a different meaning.

about from now on and that it means the same thing for all of us. Otherwise we run the risk of increasing confusion and misunderstandings.

The knowledge we have of our planet and the universe has changed dramatically in the last two centuries. What we know today about physics is totally different from what our grandparents knew. Imagine going back to the time when our ancestors were thinking about remote future scenarios of us, their heirs. It would have been impossible for them to foresee that our reality would surpass even their best fantasies. But not even in their weirdest dreams could they have foreseen what to us commonplace objects, like computer tablets are. Using their slates, they could barely write with a piece of chalk, while on today's equivalent one can watch a full-color movie with sound and even talk with people very far away and see their faces and surroundings. Some centuries ago technological progress advanced quite slowly, but now it is advancing at such a speed that it is possible for two people within the same generation to wonder about what they are witnessing. This was unthinkable a few decades earlier.

Ignoring these developments is acting like the ostrich that buries its head in the sand for fear or uncertainty, probably thinking that the not-seen threat is not a threat at all. Unintentional ignorance, which is pure or "innocent" ignorance, is not as dangerous as purposeful rejection or refusal to incorporate new or unfamiliar information, an act known as culpable ignorance[20]. In addition to any type of ignorance deviations, manipulations, and distortions have been used over time by individuals with bad intentions and obscure interests in order to manipulate fellow humans. Many of the problems we face when trying to clarify certain concepts and phenomena are due to the interference of pseudoscience and organized religions. They try to impose on us half-truths and sometimes complacent or suitable interpretations. Examples of such can be observed in writings grouped under the label of New Age, where a vocabulary pertaining to many sciences is improperly used and mixed

---

20 Culpable ignorance is the lack of knowledge or understanding that results from the omission of ordinary care to acquire such knowledge or understanding.

with superstitions and myths. Generally, in the background these texts contain undeniable truths, but what is built on top of them is impossible to be sustained. They are mostly fallacies[21], errors in reasoning in which two things that are true (assertions) are used to reach a false conclusion. Consider the following example:

- *The gold shines (true).*
- *That mirror shines (also true).*
- *Then the mirror is made out of gold (fallacy).*

Our wise ancestors coined the proverb "All that glitters is not gold," which reminds us not to be deceived by appearances or reach conclusions based on false premises.

The foregoing is important, as many people utilize the term *energy* improperly and recklessly. They say things like, "This stone has a positive energy" or "In this place I perceive a negative energy." But if we ask them a simple question—How do you define or measure that energy?—they will just babble, unable to provide a logical or coherent answer.

If we take into our hands an apple, we can touch it and even smell or taste it and also feel its temperature; therefore we know that it is a physical object composed of matter. A blind person, although unable to recall an image in his mind, may memorize a tactile sensation of any material object and recognize it afterward just by touching it. We were taught in primary school that matter can be solid, liquid, or gaseous. Even gases, which can be difficult to feel or see, are easily detected. When the wind blows, we do not see the air, but we see how objects move by its action, and we can feel its pressure on our skin and in our hair. In contrast with matter (whose characteristics are evident) energy is more difficult to specify or define, perhaps due to its invisibility and intangibility. Many texts, then, are redundant when they mention an "invisible energy." Do you know any visible one?

---

21 A fallacy is an argument that uses poor reasoning. A fallacy can be either formal or informal.

In order to further clarify this issue, let's remember that we have already an intuitive concept of energy when, for example, we express our feeling in the morning by saying, "I'm full of energy today" or "I have no energy to go to work." We also refer to others by saying, "That child has a lot of energy" or "That player lacks energy." Often the term is used as a synonym for *force*, so when we say, "I have no strength," we could express the same feeling by saying, "I have no energy." We mostly consider the terms as synonyms when referring to our own bodies. Our ancestors also had this intuitive concept of energy and realized that their physical exhaustion disappeared when they ate (replenishing their energy in chemical form) and that the cold season was better endured by sitting around a campfire (replenishing thermal energy).

"Ye shall know them by their fruits. Do men gather grapes of thorns, or figs of thistles?"[22] This religious proverb could be applied to energy, as we perceive what it is only by observing its effects on physical matter. When we see a magnet attract or repel a nail, we do not see the force of magnetic attraction but the effects that it produces; when we turn on the lights in our home, we do not see electricity flowing, but one of its effects; when we make something in a microwave oven, we are unable to see the heat that cooks our food; and when something falls down, we do not see the gravitational energy that drew it. We observe only the effects.

In our culture there is an ingrained impulse to taxonomically classify and divide everything we study. Physicists originally considered the known world around us to be composed of two basic elements: matter and energy. This preliminary division between matter and energy, which was introduced long ago, is today considered to be inaccurate due to subsequent findings in the field of nuclear energy. To modern physicists,

> The amount of matter converted into energy in the atomic bomb dropped on Hiroshima was about 700 milligrams and became an explosion equivalent to 15,000 tons of TNT.

---

22 Matthew 7:16, Christian Bible (Authorized King James Version)

making this distinction is like differentiating liquid water from ice, when they are in fact two conditions of the same element. The new physics states that matter and energy are just aspects of the same thing. Therefore in the universe, everything is energy.

In the second half of the twentieth century, research at the subatomic level showed that a threshold exists at which one cannot determine with certainty whether something is physical matter or energy. It seems that the two merge at this level, like a twilight zone where light is mixed with darkness. The new subatomic (or elementary) particles, smaller than protons and neutrons, called quarks[23], exhibit characteristics of both states. And even larger particles like photons[24]also exhibit simultaneously characteristics of both matter and energy.

In the mid-twentieth century, we witnessed for the first time the spectacular transformation of matter into energy when the atomic bomb exploded, which meant that matter could be converted into energy. The procedure was also performed in the reverse using particle accelerators that made it possible to create matter from energy using gamma-ray impacts. It should be noted that the new physics demonstrated that we see less than 10 percent of all existing matter in the universe (visible matter), since there is another stuff, invisible, they call dark matter,[25]or exotic matter, that fills out 84 percent of the cosmos.

---

23 A quark is an elementary particle and a fundamental constituent of matter. Quarks combine to form composite particles called hadrons, the most stable of which are protons and neutrons, the components of atomic nuclei.

24 Like all elementary particles, photons are currently best explained by quantum mechanics and exhibit wave-particle duality, exhibiting properties of both waves and particles. For example, a single photon may be refracted by a lens or exhibit wave interference with itself but also act as a particle, giving a definite result when its position is measured.

25 Dark matter cannot be seen directly with telescopes; evidently it neither emits nor absorbs light or other electromagnetic radiation at any significant level. Instead, its existence and properties are inferred from its gravitational effects on visible matter, radiation, and the large-scale structure of the universe. According to the Planck mission team, and based on the standard model of cosmology, the total mass-energy of the universe contains 4.9 percent ordinary matter, 26.8 percent dark matter, and 68.3 percent dark energy. Thus, dark matter is estimated to constitute 84.5 percent of the total matter in the universe.

For the purpose of this explanation, which is not the argument of a physicist nor intended for academics, let's walk the easiest track. We will continue to consider these two aspects as if they were separate, like water and ice, although we know they are the same molecular substance. Knowing that they are two aspects of the same thing can help us at certain times to understand why certain phenomena occur. So now for convenience and simplicity, we will keep this apparent division between matter and energy. We could say that in general what we call matter (mass) will be visible or perceptible, while the opposite, which is invisible and not directly perceptible, will be considered energy.

The definition that is best known in physics states, "Energy is the ability to do work." This should be read with the caveat that "work" in this context may mean something different from what it means to the average person. In some cases this concept means the same for both. When one is climbing a ladder, for instance, work equals force times distance ($W=F^*d$). But sometimes the meaning is different. One may consider holding a weight with his arms raised to be work, but because no distance displacement takes place in such an act, a physicist would say that no work is performed—only a force is exerted.

Based on the concept that energy is the ability to do work, we have to clarify a common mistake, which is attributing moral values to energy. One of the reasons many give positive or negative value to energy is that we use the term *energy* quite often as a synonym for *force*, which indeed can have a positive or negative vector value.

However, in principle energy is neither good nor evil, nor is it positive or negative. Let's consider electricity. We use it to heat food, operate the blender, raise the elevator, and so on. These are examples of good or positive outcomes. But when a criminal offender is electrocuted in the electric chair or someone accidentally touches a power line that kills him, we are talking about something bad or negative. There are a number of similar examples in which a particular energy produces either positive or negative effects. Air (aeolic energy) that turns a windmill or impels a sailboat is positive whereas a tornado or hurricane that destroys everything in its path is negative. Nuclear energy such as that of the atomic bombs dropped on Hiroshima and Nagasaki is destructive, negative, or bad. But nuclear energy that feeds electricity to a whole city or is used to cure cancer by radiation is positive or good. The possible outcomes of the use or application of energy can be good or bad, positive or negative. Most important to realize is that such outcomes depend on the intention or purpose of the one controlling the energy.

The history of civilization is intimately linked to the discovery, capture, and control of different forms of energy. In fact progress has depended on the control and domination of energy. Many different types of energy have accompanied us silently from the dawn of civilization. Consider, for example, electric energy, which has always been present in lightning bolts. People perceived as well the force of the wind's energy and that of moving water. When people put sails on their boats, they controlled the aeolic energy, which made it possible to move large vessels, and from that moment onward, humans began to use and harness the energies around them. Then humans also learned to use the energy from burning coal or wood to produce steam in boilers, which made boats and trains move faster and with more precision. Following this development, boats were fitted with combustion engines, and even many warships and submarines were equipped thereafter with nuclear-powered engines. With greater mastery and control of different energies, better results were obtained, and thus progress occurred more quickly.

Each new bit of acquired knowledge or discovery related to energy manipulation was the basis for further development. And it is significant that the progress of human civilization is closely linked to the development of energy applications. By a method of trial and error, we were evolving, beginning with the use of wind, then moving to steam, electricity, telegraph, telephone, radio, television, radar, microwaves, cell phones, computers, and smartphones, and who knows how far we can go!

By empirical observation, humans also noticed that plants deprived of sunlight did not grow. Eventually it was discovered that what made plants grow was energy, solar energy. Plants are classified as *autotrophs*, organisms that have the ability through a process known as photosynthesis to convert solar energy directly into ATP molecules and cellulose; they are virtual labs that process and store energy. This energy is indirectly transmitted to humans when they eat plants or eat meat from animals that were fed plants. Beings that are unable to directly convert solar energy are called *heterotrophs*, and we humans are among them.

Humans' ability to harness the sun's energy through plants is based on a principle known as *energy transfer*[26]. Our early ancestors were taking advantage of this principle when they sat by the fire to get warm, though they assumed that this result was due to a mysterious fluid, a conception that lasted until the late 1700s. Humans who ignored this scientific principle, and so acting empirically, applied heat transfer in their kitchens to cook, prepare, and bake their food. Then they applied it to melt metals and work on glass.

With the advancement of the sciences, especially physics, humans were able to discover a second characteristic: this energy transfer took place within a closed system, and the same amount of energy remained constant within that system. This knowledge originated from something as simple as the calculation of the amount of coal required by a steamboat or steam train. Coal was mostly used for feeding steam boilers (i.e., to produce the heat required to evaporate the water whose steam moved the engines that propelled the boat or train). To be sure that the trains or boats could operate during a specific time or across a certain distance, humans required this calculation; it provided the certainty that they would be able to complete a journey without being stranded halfway. From this activity emerged the science of thermodynamics (with *thermos* meaning "heat" and *dynamics* referring to movement). This science determined the performance of energy within the system and produced a number of laws or principles that govern it. Among the most important of these principles is the principle of conservation of energy.

---

26 Energy transfer is the transfer of energy from one object or material to another, and this is accomplished in several ways: radiation (radiant energy), heat conduction, convection, mass transfer, electrical power transmission, and mechanical work (machines).

This principle established that within a given system, energy could be transformed into another or others without being destroyed and that the total amount of energy within the system remained constant.

We have many examples of the transformation of one type of energy into another. Such happens in a chain of events when the thermal energy produced in steam boilers is converted into mechanical energy, which then makes the turbines turn to generate electrical energy. These turbines could also be propelled by the use of hydraulic, or kinetic, energy from the moving water in rivers or the descending water from lakes. The electric energy transmitted or transported to distant places is converted back into mechanical energy that drives the engine of a household blender or provides thermal energy to cook food. This reminds us that the most useful property of any energy is the ability to be transformed while maintaining its ability to perform a function. Arguably, what we understand as different energies are simply different aspects of a universal energy, an idea consistent with physicists who say that everything in the cosmos is energy.

For centuries, scientific researchers have known that energy seems to act uniformly. No exceptions have been observed in the regularity of its behavior, and this has confirmed multiple times the principle of conservation of energy. This principle is crucial to understanding the control and application of energies. Although the principle does not explain how or why this happens, scientists have established that one form of energy is exactly equivalent to another form of energy. In these transformations there are losses, usually in heat, so the resulting energy is not exactly equivalent to the original, but after the heat losses are added, the two are fully equivalent.

Radioactive substances such as uranium and thorium emit particles endowed with extraordinary energy, and Marie Curie (1867–1934) found that radium incessantly emitted heat in significant amounts, so much that a radium wave provided four thousand

> The approximate percentage of the mass of uranium atom that is converted into energy during the process of nuclear fission is 0.1.

calories per hour. None of the chemical reactions discovered up to that point was able to release even one millionth of the energy released by radium. And the amazing thing was that heat release remained hour after hour, week after week, and so for decades. In addition, that energy release was neither related nor dependent on the ambient temperature, as radium was able to release the same energy even at the lowest liquid-hydrogen temperature. This new and unusual form of energy that had nothing to do with chemical energy was labeled *nuclear energy*.

Then Albert Einstein (1879–1955) published his special theory of relativity. He showed that by mathematical calculation, mass (matter) could be considered a form of energy, which incidentally was very concentrated because a tiny amount of mass liberates an immense amount of energy. Based on his theory, Einstein produced the world's most famous equation: $e = mc^2$

This equation destroyed a sacred scientific law from the times of Lavoiser[27], the law of conservation of mass, which stated that one could not create or destroy matter. Einstein merged the conservation law of mass and that of energy (the first law of thermodynamics) into a single one: the law of mass-energy conservation. This law was expanded into the principle of conservation of mass-energy because the quantity of mass as well as that of energy in a system is conserved unless the mass is transformed into energy or a part of the energy is transformed into matter.

Just as each new discovery had been the basis for further development, current knowledge accumulated in diverse sciences such as biology, physics, and chemistry have established the foundation for the ability to scientifically determine the causes of abnormal behavior of other energies, those considered "subtle."

Having reviewed the concept of energy, we now have to mention that according to physics there are four forces (recognized and verified) that seem to govern the mechanics of the observable universe, namely

---

27 Antoine-Laurent de Lavoisier (August 26, 1743–May 8, 1794, the "father of modern chemistry," was a French nobleman prominent in the histories of chemistry and biology.

strong nuclear force, weak nuclear force, electromagnetic force, and gravitational force.

But recent decades have produced an accumulation of experimental results that cannot be explained by taking into account only these four forces and associated energies. For an explanation of these phenomena, considered anomalous, the term *subtle energy* was created. Though this type of energy still eludes examination with normal technology, it can be identified by many procedures and especially through its positive or negative effects. Subtle energy cannot be directly observed because it operates at the level of vacuum. It can be converted to observable in our present human condition only by the addition of a transducer[28]. Today, these transducers are essentially living systems.

Subtle energies explain the anomalous phenomena that cannot be accounted for by the four fundamental energies that we already know and accept. And this book is basically dealing with subtle energy and its control from an empirical point of view, which means that it is based on accumulated and unexplainable experiences around the world.

---

28 A transducer is a device that converts a signal in one form of energy to another form of energy. Energy types include (but are not limited to) electrical, mechanical, electromagnetic (including light), chemical, acoustic, or thermal energy. While the term *transducer* commonly implies the use of a sensor or detector, any device that converts energy can be considered a transducer. Transducers are widely used in measuring instruments.

CHAPTER 5

A Review of Vibration, Frequency, and Resonance

At the end of the 1800s, the reputed physicist Nikola Tesla[29]said, "If you want to find the secrets of the universe, think in terms of energy, frequency, and vibration."

Just as a clear understanding of the concept of energy is crucial, so too is an understanding of the use here of the term *vibration*. These are the two fundamental parts of what we will later describe as requirements for human control of subtle energy. Vibration (of energy) is ever present at all levels of creation, from the micro cosmos at the atomic level to the macro cosmos, where myriads of galaxies interact.

Vibration is a basic characteristic of energy. And after Albert Einstein, all modern physicists affirm that the cosmos is pure energy and that matter is just one aspect or variation of it. Being that vibration is a main characteristic of energy, we can say that the whole universe is just energy and vibration.

An ancient book named *The Kybalion: Hermetic Philosophy*[30] published in 1908 claimed to be the essence of the teachings of Hermes

---

29 Nikola Tesla (July 10, 1856–January 7, 1943) was a Serbian American inventor, electrical engineer, mechanical engineer, physicist, and futurist best known for his contributions to the design of the modern alternating current (AC) electricity supply system.

30 The *Kybalion* was first published in 1908 by the Yogi Publication Society and is now in the public domain. It can be found on the Internet.

Trismegistus, the so-called father of Hermetic knowledge. The book was published anonymously by either a group or a single person under the pseudonym of The Three Initiates. It contains seven Hermetic principles, similar to the Arcane Laws,[31] and the most important one seems to be the Third Hermetic principle, known as the Principle of Vibration, which embodies the truth that motion is manifest in everything in the universe: "Nothing rests; everything moves. Everything vibrates."

This principle, which is now supported by scientific evidence, explains that the differences between several manifestations of matter and energy are the result of different vibration levels or frequencies. Here, the *All*[32] is purported to be at an infinite level of vibration, almost to the point of being at rest. There are said to be millions upon millions of varying degrees between the highest level, the All, and the objects of the lowest vibration. The Hermetic Principle was already mentioned by some of the early Greek philosophers, who embodied it in their systems, but for centuries it was neglected by scholars outside of the Hermetic ranks. In the nineteenth century, however, physical science rediscovered this axiom, and scientific discoveries of the twentieth and twenty-first centuries added more proof of the correctness and authenticity of this ancient Hermetic doctrine.

It is surprising that such knowledge mentioned in *The Kybalion* was already known to ancient Egyptians and that people at the beginning of the twentieth century were again talking about it. Now scientists accept that the entire physical universe is made up of pure energy and

---

31 The Arcane teachings bear many superficial similarities to the *Kybalion*, The *Kybalion* explores seven Hermetic principles while the Arcane teachings examine seven Arcane laws. The *Kybalion* claims to be an elucidation of an ancient, unpublished Hermetic text of the same name while the arcane teachings claim to reveal the wisdom of an ancient, unpublished scroll of occult aphorisms. Both books describe three "great planes" of reality, which are further subdivided into seven lesser planes.

32 The *All* (also called The One, The Absolute, The Great One, The Creator, The Supreme Mind, The Supreme Good, The Father, and The Universal Mother) is the Hermetic, pantheistic view of God, which is that everything that is, or at least everything that can be experienced, collectively makes up The All. One Hermetic maxim states, "While All is in The All, it is equally true that The *All* is in *All*."

vibration. When we have the insight to see everything as vibration, the nature of the universe is revealed to us.

In the 1960s a new theory was announced to the scientific community, the Strings or Superstring theory. This theory is one of the newest upstarts in science. According to String theory, absolutely everything in the universe—all of the particles that make up matter and forces—is comprised of tiny vibrating fundamental strings. Moreover, every one of these strings is identical. The only difference between one string and another, whether it's a heavy particle that is part of an atom or a massless particle that carries light, is its resonant pattern, or how it vibrates. The theory is quite complicated and supported by nearly incomprehensible mathematical formulas that are not for us, but the interesting point is that the vibration principle has returned to be part of our frame of knowledge[33] to help us understand many phenomena.

Linked to the concept of vibration is that of *frequency*, which is defined as the number of occurrences of a repeating or cycling event per unit of time. Calculating the frequency of a repeating event is accomplished by counting the number of times that the event occurs within a specific time period, then dividing the count by the length of the time period. Therefore we are able to understand when a wheel is rotating at certain speed, like twenty cycles per second. Usually frequency is measured in Hertz (Hz)[34]. Radio stations advertise their transmitting frequency in Megahertz (Megahertz = 10^6 Hertz).

---

33 Frame of knowledge: Most people are only looking inside their own frame of knowledge. In other words they only relate to what they can see, verify, and test. They rely only on their five senses to tell them what their reality is. They are using their sensory level to define their frame of knowledge in the time we are living in. This frame, however, seems to change when science tells us that something is true. Our frame of knowledge is constantly changing since science is constantly showing us new truths. Our frame of knowledge has been changing as long as we have lived on this planet.

34 The hertz (symbol Hz) is the unit of frequency in the International System of Units (SI). It is defined as the number of cycles per second of a periodic phenomenon. One of its most common uses is the description of the sine wave, particularly those used in radio and audio applications, such as the frequency of musical tones. The unit is named for Heinrich Rudolf Hertz, who was the first to conclusively prove the existence of electromagnetic waves.

Let's summarize how vibration is ever present in our daily lives. Our mother star, the sun, emits many vibrating waves grouped into the so-called electromagnetic spectrum. Among them we can find different radio waves, microwaves, X rays, gamma rays, ultraviolet and infrared light, and finally what we call the visible spectrum of light, which is just a frequency range of vibration among which colors are simply waves vibrating at different frequencies. On one end of the spectrum is red; on the other end is violet. Red has the longest wavelength[35] and the lowest frequency; violet has the shortest wavelength and the highest frequency.

The other vibration present and noticeable in our daily lives is sound, which is made up of changes in air pressure in the form of waves. Frequency is the property of sound that most determines pitch, and people refer to different wave levels as audio frequencies. The sounds our ear can perceive are limited to a specific range of audio frequencies. Of course in this case it is not an electromagnetic vibration but air vibration. For humans, the audible range of audio frequencies is usually 20 to 20,000 Hz, although there is considerable variation among individuals, especially at high frequencies, where a gradual decline with age is considered normal. Other animals, like cats, are extremely sensitive and have the best hearing of any mammal, being most acute in the range of 500 Hz to 32 kHz. This sensitivity is further enhanced by the cat's large movable outer ears, which both amplify sounds and help a cat sense the direction from which a noise is coming. Today, we all know that dogs and cats can detect sounds that are undetectable to the human ear. When someone blows a dog whistle, we know that such a sound will be detected only by the dog.

Once we are aware of this principle and get used to thinking in terms of vibration, we can understand practically everything that happens in the physical world. This is one of the governing dynamics that allows us to make sense of everything. Vibration as it relates to energy begins with a

---

35 In physics, the wavelength (represented by the Greek letter λ, lambda) of a sinusoidal wave, is the spatial period of the wave—the distance over which the wave's shape repeats. It is usually determined by considering the distance between consecutive corresponding points of the same phase, such as crests.

microscopic atom. At the atomic level, atoms have a nucleus surrounded by tiny electrons. And there is always a subtle vibrating movement that creates a micro vibration. Since everything in the universe is made of atoms, then matter and energy are vibrational in nature.

Accelerometers and vibrometers are the instruments used to measure the vibration of any object. We are not going to discuss them in detail, but the important fact to know is that vibration is a measurable phenomenon that affects the entire universe, humans included.

It seems that all animal species communicate by vibration. Small insects like bees and crickets, among others, use specific patterns of vibration of their legs or wings to communicate. We communicate by making air vibrate with our voices at specific frequencies and tones. The human voice is specifically that part of human sound production in which the vocal folds (or vocal cords) are the primary sound source. A voice frequency or voice band is one of the frequencies within part of the audio range that is used for the transmission of speech. The voiced speech of a typical adult male will have a fundamental vibration frequency from 85 to 180 Hz, and that of a typical adult female ranges from 165 to 255 Hz. Great mammals like whales, elephants, hippopotamuses, rhinoceroses, giraffes, and alligators are known to use infrasound (ultralow frequencies) to communicate over great distances (up to hundreds of miles, in the case of whales). The study of such sound waves, sounds beneath 20 Hz down to 0.001 Hz, is called *infrasonics*. This frequency range is utilized for monitoring earthquakes and charting rock and petroleum formations below the earth. In biology these infrasonic waves are also used in seismo-cardiography to study the mechanics of the human heart.

One study has suggested that infrasound may cause feelings of awe or fear in humans. It also was suggested that since it is not consciously perceived, it may make people feel vaguely that odd or supernatural events are taking place. The presence of infrasound makes those present report anxiety, uneasiness, extreme sorrow, nervous feelings of revulsion or fear, chills down the spine, and feelings of pressure on the chest. Some scientists affirm that very low frequency sound can cause people to have unusual experiences even though they cannot consciously detect or hear the infrasound. Scientists also have suggested that this level of sound may be present at some allegedly haunted sites and so cause people to have odd sensations that they attribute to a ghost. In these events we notice that vibration is affecting humans in many ways even though we are not able to consciously perceive all of vibrating frequencies.

Both the Christian Bible and the Jewish Torah tell of a city named Jericho (Joshua 6:1–27) that was fortified with surrounding walls. It was almost impossible for the Israelites to take over that city, but by using the sound of rams' horns in coordination with human shouts to demolish a part of the wall, and they were able to penetrate the city. The story has long been considered a myth or legend by agnostics or as one of God's miracles by believers. But modern science has demonstrated that sound vibration can indeed be used as a weapon.

Sonic and ultrasonic weapons (USW) are weapons of various types that use sound to injure, incapacitate, or kill an opponent. Some sonic weapons are currently in limited use or in research and development by military and police forces. Some make a focused beam of sound or ultrasound—known as sound cannons—and others make an area field of sound. Although many sonic and ultrasonic weapons are described as nonlethal, they can still kill under certain conditions.

Cavitation[36] is a phenomena which affects gas nuclei in human tissue, and heating can result from exposure to ultrasound thus causing damage to tissue and organs. Noise-induced neurological disturbances in humans exposed to continuous low-frequency tones for durations longer than fifteen minutes have induced in some cases the development of immediate and long-term problems affecting brain tissue.

From 1983 until 1989 in Panama there was a dictator by the name of Manuel Noriega. After being toppled and removed during the US invasion of Panama, he, together with four others, took sanctuary in the

---

36 Cavitation is the formation and then immediate implosion of cavities in a liquid (bubbles or small liquid-free zones) that are the consequence of forces acting upon the liquid.

Apostolic Nunciature, (the Holy See's embassy in Panama), where he stayed some days as political refugee. The American troops, unable to take the Nunciature by force because it was the embassy of the Vatican State, decided on a harassing policy of bombardment, not with weapons, but with strong and loud acid rock broadcasted by very powerful speakers aimed at the building. After a very few days, all the people within the Nunciature were becoming sick and nearly mad from the music and agreed to deliver the dictator if the troops would stop the music.

As a consequence of being aware of the influence of different sounds on the human organism, a new science was born under the name of *psychoacoustics*.[37] Experiments and research in the field involve sound levels and sound frequencies. This science is so far advanced that some universities are offering Master's degrees[38] in that area. Many experiments have been conducted on the influence of sounds on the physiology and psychology of human beings. When hearing sounds, we can get two different feelings: the perception of the specific tone, frequency, or intensity and its correlated physiological or psychological effects.

So is the case as well with electromagnetic waves, which cannot be perceived with our five senses and nevertheless we are still subject to their influence. It is good to remember the event we can witness in a microwave when a cup of water is placed inside: the water gradually changes its temperature until it starts boiling due to the radiation of microwaves that are invisible to our naked eyes.

From this we learned that the influence of a sound or electromagnetic wave is directly proportional to a characteristic known as resonance,[39] a phenomenon directly related to vibration of any type. In the case of microwaves, these devices have a resonant frequency similar to water,

---

37 Psychoacoustics is the scientific study of sound perception. More specifically, it is the branch of science studying the psychological and physiological responses associated with sound (including speech and music).

38 Safford University in the United Kingdom is one among several.

39 In physics, resonance is the tendency of a system to oscillate with greater amplitude at some frequencies than at others. Frequencies at which the response amplitude is at a relative maximum are known as the system's resonant frequencies, or resonance frequencies.

which is present in most food components. Resonance is always related to vibration, be it mechanical, acoustical, electrical, atomic, and so forth. When we tune a TV or radio station, what we really do is use our tuning devices to search for a resonant frequency corresponding to that of the broadcasting station. Wireless communication would not be possible without resonant devices.

The existence of objects resonant to certain frequencies sometimes produces tragedies. In mechanics and construction, a *resonance disaster* describes the destruction of a building or a technical mechanism by induced vibrations at a system's resonance frequency[40], which causes it to oscillate. Broughton Suspension Bridge was one of the first suspension bridges constructed in Europe. On April 12, 1831, the bridge collapsed, reportedly due to mechanical resonance induced by troops marching over the bridge in step. As a result of the incident, the British Army issued an order that troops should break step when crossing a bridge. French soldiers were also ordered to break step on bridges; nevertheless, marching was cited as a contributing factor to the collapse of the Angers Bridge in France during a storm in 1850 in which over two hundred soldiers were killed.

It is reported that Enrico Caruso, the great Italian tenor of the early twentieth century, was the first to break a wine glass using his singing voice. Some argue that this is a myth, but modern science considers it possible provided that certain circumstances were present. Wine glasses, because of their hollow shape, are particularly resonant. If you run a damp finger along the rim of a glass, you might hear a faint, ghostly humming, which is the resonant frequency of the glass. Caruso's pitch and that of the fragile wine flute likely had the same resonant frequency. Furthermore tenors usually sing at high-intensity levels, which means

---

40 Mechanical resonance is the tendency of a mechanical system to absorb more energy when the frequency of its oscillations matches the system's natural frequency of vibration than it does at other frequencies. It may cause violent swaying motions and even catastrophic failure in improperly constructed structures, including bridges, buildings, trains, and aircraft. When designing objects, engineers must ensure the mechanical resonance frequencies of the component parts do not match driving vibrational frequencies of motors or other oscillating parts, a phenomenon known as resonance disaster.

Caruso should have sung at a sound level exceeding 105 decibels[41]. These two factors could allow one to break a glass with just his or her voice. Another surprising effect of resonance was reported in a very famous case of political espionage conducted by Russians in the US embassy in Moscow in the early 1950s. This event is known as the "Great Seal bug story"[42] and was performed using resonant frequencies of certain devices placed inside.

Resonance phenomena occur with all types of vibrations or waves: there is mechanical resonance, acoustic resonance, electromagnetic resonance, nuclear magnetic resonance, electron spin resonance, and resonance of quantum wave functions. Resonant systems can be used to generate vibrations of a specific frequency (e.g., musical instruments). Some of the phenomena we are going to discuss could be partly explained by the *Morphic Resonance*[43] thought to occur in living beings.

I am trying to mostly avoid technicalities; they can be further investigated by interested parties. But so far I hope to have clarified the following important concepts: systems, energy, vibration, and resonance, all of them closely intertwined and very helpful in understanding some extraordinary phenomena associated with human beings.

---

41 A decibel (dB) is one tenth of a bel, a seldom-used unit named in honor of Alexander Graham Bell. It is a logarithmic unit used to express the ratio between two values of a physical quantity (usually measured in units of power or intensity). The decibel is used for a wide variety of measurements in science and engineering, most prominently in acoustics, electronics, and control theory.

42 In 1946, Soviet schoolchildren presented a two-foot wooden replica of the Great Seal of the United States to Ambassador Averell Harriman. The ambassador hung the seal in his office in Spaso. During George F. Kennan's ambassadorship in 1952, a secret technical surveillance countermeasures (TSCM) inspection discovered that the seal contained a wireless microphone with a resonant cavity that could be stimulated from an outside radio signal.

43 Morphic Resonance theory was introduced by Alfred Rupert Sheldrake, stating that memory is inherent in nature and that certain living structures are able to capture information from their kind fellows living in the past or at remote distances and modify their biological characteristics and performance accordingly. See *Morphic Resonance: The Nature of Formative Causation* by Rupert Sheldrake (Park Street Press, 2009).

CHAPTER 6

Cathay

Anthropologists, paleontologists, and archaeologists base their careers, lives, and studies on discoveries of ancient remains—structures or objects that have been hidden or inaccessible for centuries. Those objects, ruins, monuments, documents, and temples stayed in their original place, waiting to be found in a future time. In many cases their previous existence was unknown, and findings were incidental or unexpected; in other cases hints were obtained from old legends and historical or religious accounts.

In the imperial and feudal lords' time, China's inhabitants believed that their country was the center of the world. Due to the country's large geographic area and different topographies, ancient Chinese culture was traditionally a closed society. The diverse inhabitants, including members of fifty-six different ethnic groups, were eventually merged, after the Warring States period (475–221 BC), as China gradually began to form a vast empire. At that time there was very little contact with the outside world. Any contact was usually made through trade mostly made through the Silk Road, originally a way for camel caravans to cross the Taklimakan Desert in Western China to reach the Middle East and Arabia. Subsequently a trade route was established by sea that also linked China with the Middle East. Through these routes the Chinese exported silk and jade while bartering for other goods. These routes also initiated a social and religious exchange.

China's isolation from other cultures was also evident in the internal remoteness among provinces or towns belonging to different kingdoms, which resulted in the creation of multiple languages or dialects. Currently in China there are still 205 living languages, and they still hold some 1,800 dialects. The Mandarin language, from the Han-dominant ethnic group, is now China's common or standard language (Putonghua)[44]; it was imposed as the national official language only after the revolution in 1949.

The Chinese were among the first intrepid travelers, often risking their lives to venture into the Silk Road. Their unchallenged hero was Zhang Qian, whom Emperor Wu Di, of the Han dynasty, sent to the West in 139 BC to build alliances against the Xiongnu, traditional enemies of the Chinese. However, the Xiongnu captured Zhang Qian and imprisoned him. Thirteen years later, he escaped and returned to China. The emperor, who appreciated the richness of detail and accuracy of Zhang Qian's reports, sent him to visit several neighboring nations in the year 119 BC. The successful mission paved the way for the future ambassadors and travelers between East and West.

Buddhism spread to China, and several Chinese Buddhist monks made pilgrimages to India to bring sacred texts. Their traveling diaries are an extraordinary source of information. For example, the journal of Fa Xian (describing fourteen years travel, between 399 and 414 AD) made a substantial contribution to our knowledge of the history of Central Asia during the fifth century. The journal of Xuan Zang (spanning twenty-five years, between 629 and 654) has an enormous historical value as well and inspired a sixteenth-century comedic novel, *Pilgrimage to the West*, which became one of the most important Chinese classics. During the Middle Ages, monks and European traders traveled in the opposite direction.

---

44 The common national speech of Han nationality using Beijing pronunciation as the standard pronunciation, using Beijing speech as the basic dialect, and using the model writing of the modern vernacular prose as the norm of grammar, is called **Putonghua.**

The first Western contact with China, formerly known in Europe as Cathay,[45] occurred circa 1266 AD. At that time, the emperor Kublai Khan, of Mongol origin, learned that some Latino aliens (of Latium) had entered his territory. He sent delegates to meet them and bring them to the capital city in order to learn something about the world outside his borders. These foreigners were Maffeo and Nicolo Polo, father and uncle of the famous Marco Polo. They had entered the Chinese empire by mistake while trying to return to Venice from Turkey by using another way eastward to avoid war zones. Years later they returned to China, this time accompanied by Marco (1254–1324), who was sixteen years old and who then remained in China for twenty-four years. Marco and his relatives arrived in the capital of the empire in the year 1275 (soon after the Eighth Crusade). There he held positions of consideration, including adviser to Kublai Kahn, and as he approached his death, he returned to Venice and had the opportunity to narrate his experiences. The knowledge of gunpowder, paper, paper money, asbestos, and more was due to his stories and experiences, although many of his contemporaries did not believe him and so nicknamed him *Il Millione* because according to them he had told a million lies. Later historians determined the veracity of most of his reports.

Until the early 1980s, information about China was scarce and mysterious. We just knew it was a very large country with a large population and that its system of government was Communist. At that time, Mao Zedong (Mao Tse-tung) was a legend, and because of the Cold War, any information about China that reached us was distorted and generally negative. The Chinese isolation during the Cold War was called the Bamboo Curtain, compared to the Iron Curtain of the Communist countries in Eastern Europe. With the changes in China

---

45 Originally, Cathay was the name applied by Central and Western Asians and Europeans to northern China; for centuries Cathay and China were believed by Europeans to be distinct nations with distinct cultures. However, by the late 1600s, Europeans had mostly become aware that these were in fact the same nation.

and the rise to power of Deng Xiaoping[46], the country began a reforming period, which allowed us from that time to know more about Chinese culture; reciprocally it allowed the Chinese to know a little more about the outside world.

In the last decades, changes in China have been dramatic and growth has been explosive, but before that, direct trade with China was very poor due to a political blockage that favored the United Kingdom: the only way of trading was through Hong Kong, a city that was still a British colony and the overseas exit door for most Chinese products.

My first contact with and travel to China was mainly commercial, as the company I was working for bought metal-working machinery in Shanghai. To keep track of deliveries and the quality of these machines, I made my first trip to China in 1989, accompanied by the commercial counselor of the embassy in my country, Mr. Luo Liecheng. In order to find new suppliers for industrial products, the two of us toured for a month the Chinese territory from Guangzhou (Canton), in the extreme south, to the northern city of Mudanjiang in the province of Heilongjiang, near the Russian border. The tour included Wuxi (Jiangsu Province), Shanghai, Nanjing (Jiangsu Province), Beijing, Changchun (Jilin Province), and Harbin (Heilongjiang Province), among other cities. It was an unforgettable experience and a clash between two cultures and worldviews. Although at that time there were still many restrictions on foreigners, we enjoyed the courtesy, hospitality, and friendship that was offered to us, which reminded me of Marco Polo. I did not expect at that time that I would be returning to that country nearly every year during more than twenty-five years.

Shortly after returning to my country from that first voyage, I went to the commercial office of the Chinese embassy to meet a friend after he had just finished doing some exercises in the garden of the residence that was assigned to him as counselor. At that moment, I perceived him

---

46 Deng Xiaoping (August 22, 1904–February 19, 1997) was a politician and reformist leader of the Communist Party of China who, after Mao's death, led his country toward a market economy. He served as the "paramount leader" of the People's Republic of China from 1978 to 1992.

as quite different: his face was radiant, he looked very well and was very energetic, there was a sense of power in his closeness, his eyes shone, and he appeared to be larger and stronger than he actually was. I was surprised. Usually after completing an exercise, one looks tired, sweaty, and exhausted, but he didn't. This encounter made me curious; I wanted to know why upon finishing his exercises he looked more energetic and radiant instead of less. I asked him what type of exercise he had practiced, to which he replied that it was called Qigong (Chi-Kung). This was my first encounter with that kind of knowledge.

After having seen the effects that this practice produced in the Chinese counselor, I thought it might be good for me to practice these exercises as well. Intrigued, I started my own brief research on the subject. My business activities allowed me scant free time; my friend's time was similarly limited. Because he did not have the opportunity to give me more detailed information, I thought it best to ask another Chinese friend of mine, Mr. Yaoming Xu, about this topic.

Yaoming, who had been representative of Xinhua, the news agency of China, gave me more information because he had friends who were masters of Qigong, and he even offered me to put me in touch with one of them. With the information he provided, I learned that Qigong is an art or science with a very ancient tradition in China. He also told me many anecdotes and narrated extraordinary events attributed to Qigong masters, events that some would consider myths or fables. Qigong had been a cultivated knowledge that was transmitted by two channels. The first was the monastery, where disciples learned from experienced senior monks. The second, outside the monasteries, were masters who taught their children, usually the firstborn male, establishing a lineage that perpetuated teachings from generation to generation. However, not all Chinese were certain about the results and power of Qigong, and many considered it a superstition.

The existence of Qigong began to be disclosed to the West, generally by overseas Chinese (Taiwanese and Cantonese) immigrants, but that teaching was misunderstood and thus regarded as a fashionable training method within the body-building market. Although many people confuse the name with some of the martial arts, Qigong is not a traditional form of exercise. It is more an art or science based on the controlling and emission of a universal energy known to the Chinese as qi (气). Qi can be applied in various fields, the martial arts being only one. This art or science is detached from any religious belief and so I consider it one of the best approaches to control subtle energy.

CHAPTER 7

A Controlling System— What Is Qigong?

(**Simplified Chinese:** 气功; **traditional Chinese:** 氣功)

Explaining a method to control and enhance subtle energy is not simple because we are speaking of controlling something invisible and intangible. Furthermore, it is a concept that could be culturally biased. But let's start by making a comparison. Suppose a native has been moved from the Amazon jungle to any of our modern cities. There he faces a number of devices and objects that although part of our daily routine, for him are something new, strange, innovative, and awesome. Take, for example, one of the simplest objects—the cell phone. As he looks at this unusual object, certain questions will arise in his mind, and surely he will demand clarification. The first question would be, "What is it?" We would of course reply that it is a device called a "telephone." He might take it in his hands to touch and even smell it, which is an identification process. Then he would make a second question: "What is it used for?" And we would explain that such device is used to talk to people who are far away. That would be something difficult for him to grasp because until this point he was unable to reach anyone outside the reach of his shouts. Talking to someone in another city would be unbelievable. But upon accepting that possibility, he generates another question.

"How is it used?" he would ask. We would explain that the handset should be placed close to the ear and that he should press a few buttons with his hand in order to get in touch with a distant person. Having overcome the initial fear and after understanding our explanations, he would be able to use the equipment efficiently. So far he has managed to acquire empirical knowledge, by which one can use objects and perform actions to achieve results without knowing the technicalities or the system that generates such results. In our own history we can observe a sequence of events in which humans initially managed to make use of many procedures, sometimes accompanied by rituals, to obtain desired results without knowing their origin or cause. The time it takes to be able to manage or get acquainted with certain procedures can take from a week to some years. But finding out and understand the underlying mechanism that produces the desired outcome could take longer—even centuries.

After being able to grasp the procedure, in this case to use the phone, our aboriginal acquires the empirical knowledge to use it advantageously. Any further question, like, "How does it function?" is irrelevant to his taking advantage of its use. And such a question would be very difficult to answer because it requires prior specialized knowledge. Thus the process likely remains a secret, and this unrevealed information could mean magical origins for him. In fact, it is not necessary for us to look for natives in the deep jungle to illustrate this point. There are plenty of people in our modern cities who do not know the technicalities of their phones; still, despite their ignorance, they regularly use them to communicate, play games, and take pictures.

Having empirical knowledge means having the skill or the capacity to use something. This could range from reading a simple in-box instruction to studying a thick handbook or even participating in courses and training seminars. Answering the question of how to use something can take months for a trained pilot when he changes the type of airplane he is flying, and if he has to start from scratch, it will take years. For this we have created a term in English that has been adopted internationally: *know-how*, or expertise. This know-how has become a money-making product in itself, and although it is intangible, it has an accounting and trade value. It can be transferred, sold, purchased, used under license, and shared. Know-how in general does not include the origin or technicalities, as those like Grandma's secret recipes, are supposed to be jealously guarded. There are some who are proud and willing to share their knowledge, but others avoid doing so for fear of losing certain dominant positions. In other cases certain knowledge or expertise is only partially transferred; the owner keeps a portion secret (e.g., a chemical formula), which forces or induces the user to purchasing commitments. The current system known as *franchising* implies the use and transfer of certain know-how, and there are even international treaties to protect what is known as intellectual property.

What arouses our interest in certain objects, devices, or procedures is their advantageous application, their ability to benefit us. Usually people think about the usefulness of an object or tool and determine whether it is worth the cost. Then they can advance to the next step, which is acquiring the object and learning the method or procedure to use it. But it is precisely in this analysis stage that the seeds of deception can be planted by assigning maliciously false properties to the announced product or action. Here reside the roots of scams, in which people are induced to acquire something based on proclaimed properties that are merely a hook to make a profit at the expense of others' ignorance. This is valid for material objects or products and as well as intangible methods, procedures, and the like.

How many people who suffer from baldness have been deceived more than once by miraculous products that supposedly will recover their lost hair? How many have been deceived with aphrodisiacs or slimming products? How many have been deceived by purported panaceas? How many have been scammed by fanciful investments? Some deceiving offers could be just a waste of time and money, but regretfully there are cases in which deception can bring very undesirable and irreversible physical or mental consequences.

In relation to procedures on how to use something, historically when humans had access to something unusual but useful, they sought to use it to their advantage. We see this quite frequently today with material goods, but it occurred as well in the development of our civilization any time an individual took advantage of empirical knowledge of certain procedures, rituals, and mental states that allowed him or her to do things that his or her peers could not and used that knowledge to dominate or control the surrounding human beings.

Unfortunately even today the knowledge of something supposedly extraordinary grants holders a kind of power over their ignorant fellows. In ancient Japan simple things like metallurgy or manufacturing a steel sword were strictly guarded secrets and transmitted only to the adepts after a rigorous selection process. Manufacturing processes were not made public and were accompanied by songs and supposedly magical formulas. In our modern industrialized world, patents protect the owners of manufacturing processes to prevent them from becoming widespread. On the nonmaterial side, several forms of subtle energy control in ancient cultures gave rise to the esoteric part of many organized religions.

When a monkey or a dog meets with someone it doesn't know, it stops and stares at the person. The dog may bark if it does not like the person; the monkey may go backward, out of sight, trying to observe the intruder from a distance. A man in the same situation will communicate with words and ask questions that will determine his reaction. Fortunately our species has the ability to communicate verbally and in that way get information and learn new things to continue evolving. Although many of our questions have a simple answer—what's your name? Who are you? What do you want?—other questions are not that simple to answer or have no answer at all. Consider, for example, what does a lemon taste like? When I first heard about Qigong (that so far was unknown to me and to the people I usually was in contact with), I began asking myself questions whose answers just led to a supplementary question, or to a black box. I also conducted research in books. Some of them were quite good, others were second-rate, and many were just trash, but I tried getting the most out of all of them.

For us Westerners, the discovery of a system to control subtle energy, like the Chinese Qigong, is similar to primitive aborigines' discovery of fire's properties and the way to control it at will. They used it but did not know its origin, and this gave fire a magical character that endured for many centuries.

Many of the phenomena observed in the practice and application of Qigong seem also to defy logic. It is not presumed that an ax blow to the chest will do no harm or that a little-known technique can provide healing that could not be achieved by traditional methods. Nor it is logical to foresee events in a distant place or future time or to capture other people's thoughts telepathically. Those events are considered extraordinary, paranormal, or metaphysical because their explanation is beyond or outside the boundaries of what is considered normal.

When we finally become aware that there are indeed many existing truths that have been hidden from us, many of us face a problem because our cultural or social patterns and our preconceived values clash with those of the alien culture. There are many who suddenly change from white to black, from light to darkness, without understanding that there are intermediate shades of gray and threshold light. In my continued studies of Qigong, I had a great advantage: paradoxically, the fact of not being Chinese. I mention this because I can take a critical and independent point of view without being attached to any fanaticism, and from this position I can understand that much of the knowledge that is provided by Qigong is not exclusive. It is shared by other disciplines and cultures, albeit with different names. Although in the past Qigong was a secret discipline, I should acknowledge the advantage of modern Qigong, which exists within a different framework, one without any religious-sectarian rituals.

There is a fable, or possibly a true story, attributed to an ancient Chinese master named Pai Chang (who lived during the Tang dynasty) narrating that he ordered some of his disciples who wanted to learn the art of Qigong to go searching for wild oxen in the open fields. Many returned saying that they had found none, and the master sent them back home. One of the disciples succeeded in locating one and informed the master, who said, "Catch it and tame it so you can ride on it." The disciple did not understand what this action could have to do with his desire to learn Qigong, but faithful to the tradition of Chinese obedience, he did what his master ordered. After he completed the task, his master clearly explained him his logic. Searching for the wild ox was a first step, he explained, like searching for qi (i.e., perceiving, feeling, and differentiating it). But it wasn't enough: the disciple also had to control it, which was like taming the wild ox and learning to ride it. People cannot control something they do not know. But simply knowing will not do us much good. We must subdue the subtle energy as humans dominated water, fire, electricity, and nuclear power.

As a business representative of a corporation based in Nanjing (capital of the Chinese province of Jiangsu) I have been traveling to China on a regular basis since 1989, which has allowed me to collect firsthand information on Qigong and to have personal contact with some masters. I experienced a change from being just a curious man to a frantic student of the subject, which later on allowed me to humbly reach a higher level. The information previously available and many of the written stories about Qigong in our Western languages were transmitted by Chinese people from mainland China, Taiwanese people, or people from Hong Kong (Xiānggǎng).

In many of the available books on this subject, the authors, just to satisfy their arrogance and narcissism, have created many different names for supposed varieties of Qigong. In books written by Westerners, the authors present Qigong as a great discovery, and each of the authors considers himself or herself a successful explorer. Unfortunately, such writers only show one side of the coin, omitting anything that is common to other cultures. Sometimes they even adopt a more fanatical attitude than Chinese nationals.

Human beings have the tendency to pay more attention to results than to the hard work required to achieve them. A friend of mine says that planting a seed is voluntary, but the harvest is compulsory. As the Bible remind us in Galatians 6:7, "God is not mocked, for whatever one sows, that will he also reap."

We should not neglect those experiences transmitted to us by previous generations. Often they are the basis for research. Further, we must be respectful while studying the past. China and India have thousands of years of culture and written history that has unfortunately been distorted by the Western point of view.

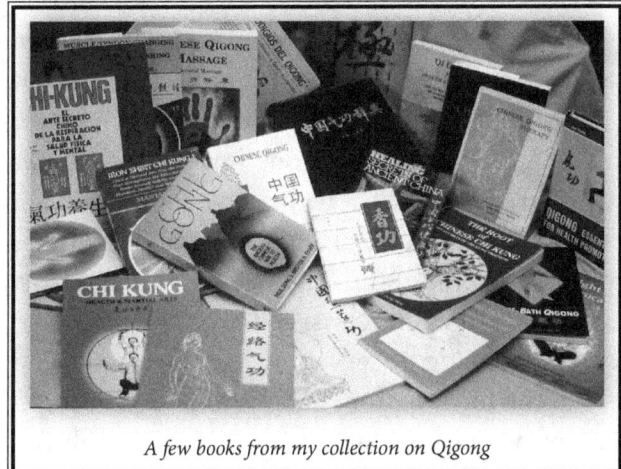

A few books from my collection on Qigong

In the past, Qigong was considered by many to be one more of those superstitions that were inherited over time or as a collection of myths. At one point this came to worry the Chinese government that took power during the revolution in 1949. To my understanding, they had reason to worry. Superstitions are harmless until they become dogmas and force people to believe in them, and such a process could have eventually undermined the unity of the Chinese nation. The ruling Communist party, to dispel the Qigong myth or superstition (that was considered, like religions, to be the opium of the people), ordered several scientific institutes and universities to investigate the phenomena related to Qigong. Despite some inconsistencies in the results, possibly by preconditioning or bias of the researchers, a large majority of the phenomena attributed to Qigong were evident, verifiable, and repeatable in the laboratory. So from that point onward, the practice could not be discredited, even though it could not be explained rationally. Qigong became the subject of serious scientific study, and regarded as a science or an art, that was free of any religious attachment or connotation. It is now a formal science, and as such has its own methods, a body of theories, experiments with results evidencing the hypotheses, an objective and a vast literature, which in the Chinese language alone has over seven thousand books published. This is not peanuts!

Is Qigong really a science using scientific methods? Or is it a protoscience, on its way to being established as a sound scientific discipline? For any area of knowledge to be considered a science, it needs a body of techniques for investigating phenomena, acquiring new knowledge, or correcting and integrating previous knowledge. So far it seems Qigong fulfills these requirements. To be termed scientific, a method of inquiry must be based on empirical and measurable evidence subject to specific principles of reasoning, and Qigong has both. The only problem with Qigong (and why we could classify it as a protoscience) is that in spite of following systematic observation, measurement, and experiment, it is still missing the formulation, testing, and modification of hypotheses, the latter of which is due to the difficult subject. Nonetheless, its effects are known, verified, and replicated.

We are bound to empirical knowledge, not so different from our ancestors when they started to use fire without knowing why it was burning. Scientific researchers propose hypotheses as explanations of phenomena and design experimental studies to test these hypotheses via predictions that can be derived from them. These steps must be repeatable in order to guard against mistake or confusion by any particular experimenter. The closest approach to explain Qigong thus far is the theory of controlling subtle energy, and the scientific community has not reached an agreement on this theory.

Scientific inquiry is generally intended to be as objective as possible in order to reduce biased interpretations of results. Another basic expectation is that researchers will document, archive, and share all data and methodology, making this information available for careful scrutiny by other scientists who can then verify results by attempting to reproduce trials. In this regard Qigong researchers and practitioners have produced a huge amount of documentation in several languages, including statistical measurements on the reliability of these data. Due to the fact that Qigong encompasses different domains, such as medicine, extrasensory perception, and bodily strengthening applied to martial arts, it is now intermingled with other sciences, and their results contribute to clarify the origins and characteristics of the subtle energy qi.

So far Qigong has been able to fulfill some of the requirements of the scientific method, like *replication*, which means that if an experiment cannot be repeated to produce the same results, this implies that the original results were an error. But so far most of the outcomes of Qigong have been replicated to a point at which there is no doubt about their veracity, and furthermore these results coincide with unrelated experiments on similar phenomena conducted in reputed international institutions.

Also Qigong has been submitted to external review. The process of peer review, involving evaluation of experiments by experts, allows for unbiased criticism. It does not certify correctness of the results, only that the experiments themselves were sound. Qigong researchers also participate in data recording and sharing in a very precise way in order to reduce their own bias and aid in replication by others who wish to verify any results.

Elements of the scientific method followed by researchers and people who practice Qigong include observation, definition, measurements, description, characterization, prediction, experiments, analysis, and explanation.

As previously mentioned, Qigong is not the only method used to control subtle energy, but it has the advantage of not being tied up with any religious beliefs or rituals, and the coverage of its applications are wider than any other single method. Qigong gives us certain powers and abilities or increases our natural gifts, but our personal effort is essential. That is why some authors say that the correct definition of Qigong is "training or study on the Qi that requires long time and great effort"

CHAPTER 8

What Is It Good For?

A friend of mine, Ms. Huan Xiu Hong (Josephine), who worked for the Chinese corporation that I represented, mentioned that she had long ago served as an interpreter for a group of foreign medical students interested in acupuncture, an opportunity that allowed her to meet one university professor who practiced and studied the control of vital energy (qi). Now retired, he'd worked on the faculty of pure sciences in the school of physics at Nanjing University. His specialty was the control and study of qi energy. (In Western terms he would be a professor of physics, specializing in the control of subtle energy). This professor was also a renowned Qigong master, and because of my interest in that area, I told Josephine that I would like to meet him in person.

Josephine was kind enough to invite Professor Tian Sheng Wu to the corporate headquarters of the company, where we could meet. After introductions and polite questions, we address the issue of his specialty, qi, and I told him about my concerns, research, and

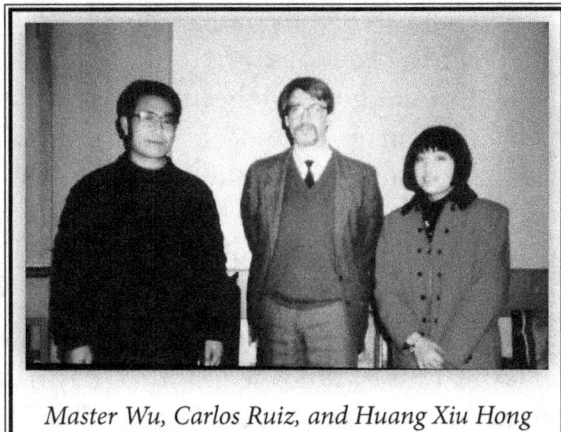

Master Wu, Carlos Ruiz, and Huang Xiu Hong

practice. I explained that I had noticed in my research that the concept that they, the Chinese, have of qi coincides with the Hindu concept of prana in India and that other cultures in different periods have given it different names, making it a universal knowledge.

I informed him as well that I had just started practicing Qigong exercises. He listened attentively and asked me some questions through Ms. Huan, including one in which he said he was intrigued about how far I had progressed in the practice of controlling the subtle energy with Qigong. He proposed a simple assessment test.

To conduct this test, the master asked me to get up from the chair and walk a distance of approximately seven meters (twenty-one feet) to the far end of the conference room. He asked me to turn around and remain relaxed. When I was in the right place, I felt as if some force had pushed me against the wall, but I felt no physical contact acting upon me; it was something more like a magnetic force. I managed to stay in balance with great effort and immediately turned back. I saw Master Wu Tian with a slight smile on his lips and Ms. Huang with a look of astonishment. The master had made a gentle movement with the palm of his hand pointing at me, yet this imperceptible movement must have activated something that impelled me hard despite the physical separation.

He explained what he was able to determine from what had just taken place: my level of qi was pretty good, but "it had not gone enough down the legs" (a comment I did not understand). He further clarified that if my level had been lower, I probably would have hit the wall in front of me and would not have been able to maintain my balance as I in fact had. I was unable to understand that event in rational terms based on what I knew about basic physics, applied force, or the principle of action and reaction, but whether I could explain it or not, I had experienced it. Ancient Chinese literature indicates that in many instances masters made their disciples or opponents fly through the air with a simple hand gesture, and although these stories always seemed far-fetched and fantastic, I now acknowledged that they had some degree of credibility, omitting, of course, exaggerations added during oral transmission.

The anomalous actions executed by Qigong masters reminded me of our Western chronicles, particularly the hagiographies (reports on the miracles of the Catholic saints), which are documented cases in which people flew through the air, possibly due to the same force. Such was the case with St. Theresa of Avila, who was said that her fellow nuns had to grab her garment to lower her down to the ground when she floated between them; the case of St. Joseph of Cupertino (1663), who was seen flying countless times and even managed the conversion to Christianity of the Duke of Brunswick, who, puzzled, observed the phenomenon. The known medium Douglas Home (1852) also levitated before countless witnesses from a lower floor to the upper floor.

Tibetan monastic schools known as 'Lung-Gom' used to train their messengers in a breathing method combined with a kind of buoyant levitation during altered states of consciousness that allowed them to cover long distances at good speed by not feeling the weight of their own bodies. Pilgrims in Tibet took three days to walk around the periphery of Mount Kailash, but they were surpassed by the *Lung-Gom-Pa* runners,[47] who made the journey in just one day. The Marathon monks of Japan, Kaihōgyō (回峰行), are quite similar to these runners of old Tibet. Many records describe these amazing running Japanese monks who appear to fly when they run. They seem to float, apparently in a trance. They are said to travel nonstop for forty-eight hours or more and can cover more than one hundred miles a day. Many are said to be faster than horses. The famous Buddhist monk Milarepa was often seen floating in the air as did St. Teresa and St. Joseph of Cupertino. In the tradition of Islam, many cases of Sufi masters have been reported, individuals who also have levitated, and the modern Transcendental Meditation TM ® in their

---

47   The word *Lung*, pronounced [*rlun*], signifies the state of air as well as vital energy or psychic force. *Gom* means meditation, contemplation, or concentration of mind and soul upon a certain subject. A lung-gom-pa runner is not a man who has the ability to fly through air, but one who can control his energy, rechannel and concentrate it in a new direction.

courses on *shiddis*[48] (or superhuman powers) produce this phenomenon (a procedure already described in the *Yoga Sutras* of Patanjali).

There are several schools of Qigong, depending on the different groups that are united by their religious or philosophical concept. Generally modern Qigong is detached from any religious connotation, but the religious groups or philosophical currents that were already established continue to include it as part of their ancestral traditions. So the followers of Confucius, the Taoists, and Buddhists practice it. However, two schools stand out in the eyes of the public for showing the most amazing and visible effects. The first is the medical school, which is more pragmatic and concerned with the therapeutic applications for healing the body and which surprises many with its miraculous cures. It is not linked to any precise philosophical or religious group, though some of these groups share this application procedure. The second is *Wushu*, a Chinese martial art aimed at physical strengthening for defense and combat, which undoubtedly is the demonstration that has caused more interest and admiration.

Regardless of which school includes qigong as a part of its studies or training, the specific branches of application that all of them share are as follows:

1. **First application: preventive Qigong**. This type does not change anything but creates the conditions for a better life. So the objective is to live longer, be healthier and be more active by practicing certain exercises.
2. **Second application: Qigong for strength and martial arts**. This type seeks to strengthen the defense and physical combat skills. Note that these capacities are not achieved overnight; they require extensive and hard physical training combined with mental conditioning.

---

48 *Siddhi* is a Sanskrit noun that can be translated as "perfection," "accomplishment," "attainment," or "success." A siddhi may be any unusual skill or faculty or capability. In Hinduism eight siddhis (*ashta Siddhi*) are known.

3. **Third application: therapeutic Qigong.** This is basically the most reputed application because is related to everyone's health. In China it is studied in medicine faculties and is mostly applied by physicians, though some reputed masters apply some of the techniques. At this point I must insert a warning: Qigong in its therapeutic application (LIAO-FA) is not intended in any way to substitute or replace conventional treatments and medical prescriptions. On the contrary, in many cases, it is an adjuvant, helping, or accessory treatment. But always it is at the discretion of the physician to implement it alone or combined with traditional medicine.

4. **Fourth application: paranormal (extrasensory) Qigong.** Another interesting type, this is also the most mysterious and secretive because it involves the generation, development, and increasing of paranormal abilities, such as telepathy, clairvoyance, premonitions, clairaudience, telekinesis, and remote viewing. Although many myths have been created around this type of Qigong, all contain a certain degree of veracity and are based on true experiences.

Some scholars include **a fifth application** they call *spiritual enlightenment*, which is usually practiced in monasteries.

All these applications have in common the control of subtle energy (qi) to achieve intended goals or objectives. Although basically Qigong involves qi gathering, it is not advisable to accumulate excess qi, which is just as damaging as a deficiency. For a graphic example of this warning, imagine trying to connect a TV directly to the high-voltage lines at a power-transmission tower. Chances are the person cannot even approach the tower before being struck by a discharge. It is the same power that feeds the TV in the house or the kitchen, but the house is limited to 110 or 220 volts while transmission lines can carry from 23,000 to 550,000 Volts. This example also serves to remind us that working with energies of any kind can be very dangerous when their properties are not fully known. In general, excess or imbalanced energy completely changes effects. We looked at the example of electricity, but the world is full of such scenarios: hydraulic energy is good for moving generating turbines to produce electricity, but that force present in rivers during flooding periods destroys everything in its way. The wind (Aeolic energy) is needed to freshen up, but we do not want to have hurricanes, typhoons, and tornadoes. The extreme cold freezes us, extreme heat transforms green fields into deserts—the list is endless.

It is not the primary objective of Qigong to develop paranormal powers or extrasensory perceptions. However, these tend to be increased automatically as a collateral effect when one conducts exercises to promote the flow of qi. Only at higher levels are drills and exercises conducted with the specific purpose of developing one or more paranormal powers.

About the use of certain unusual powers, I remember Master Wu, who told me that we should not feel different or special due to the powers that we acquire with the study of Qigong or any other system of controlling subtle energy. That advice, in Western terms, means to avoid infatuation. These events just make us aware of what we can achieve or, more accurately, what we must awaken in us, since we were born with it. Some people, unfortunately, take advantage of these effects to gain followers whom they exploit and subjugate while they proclaim themselves masters or gurus. But on the other side are conscious humans who become aware of their psychic powers and do not consider themselves any different; they understand that these experiences and powers are not unusual, but inherent and innate to human nature and that they are shared as well by animals and even plants.

CHAPTER 9

How Does It Function?

How does this procedure function? That was the first question I asked myself when I began studying Qigong. My first searches for an explanation were frustrating. Many books that claimed full coverage of the issue dealt superficially with just one of the aspects, and most of them sold the idea of a new series of exotic gymnastic exercises. In addition to reading multiple books, I watched some videos as well, but those, too, fell short. Instead of being a help, they just introduced confusion, suggesting that by repeating like a robot some movements or positions shown on the screen, one would achieve something. Due to experienced frustration sometimes Qigong gets a bad reputation and well-intended students finally quit practicing because they did not obtain any benefit, ignoring that what they watched is only a portion of a much larger body of knowledge.

After overcoming many difficulties and misunderstandings, some people can get a clearer idea of what Qigong is, but understanding something does not necessarily mean one can use or apply it. Physicians in medical schools study a lot of theory, but they cannot become true and effective doctors until they begin practicing. This applies to pilots, engineers, and in general all professions. In our daily life, we move from a passive or theoretical knowledge into practice in order to master any art or craft.

But there are cases in which some training cannot be completed due to physical limitations or other hindrances. Many pilots would like to be astronauts, but most cannot. Many men understand perfectly the fertilization process and subsequent intrauterine growth of infants, but they cannot get pregnant, as pregnancy is reserved only for women. Many coaches know how to do something and explain it so that an athlete can achieve a higher level of performance, but often they are unable to do it by themselves. Qigong, like any art or science, has a theoretical basis and a practicing system. Studying it is like entering a school of music or any other artistic activity: one should first learn the basic theory and principles of that art. With time, practice combined with talent can yield great performers or artists. The study of Qigong, like the study of many other arts and sciences, guarantees equal opportunity—not equal results.

The Homo sapiens species has evolved through a constant process of learning and mastering new techniques. Since the dawn of civilization, this process was based largely on observations and attempts based on trial and error. Observation is essential to learning anything, and we tend to focus our observations on anything that is strange or unusual. In this way we can use and apply what we discovered or simply avoid any hazard or keep away from dangerous situations. For example, in the remote past, humans avoided predators after having observed a beast attacking and then devouring a small animal. Primitive humans observed that fire burned and destroyed whatever it came in contact with. After extinguishing the flames, they also noticed that the site where fire had been burning remained completely hot. They concluded from these observations that the fire could serve to warm them on cold days and nights. They also noticed that at night the fire produced light that could be used to see in the darkness even though the sun was not present.

Observation is not always a passive activity. Often it leads to a verification process by trial and error that involves taking a risk. For example, the man next to a campfire realized that it was warmer near the fire. Possibly he or someone else, moved by curiosity, tried to put his hand in the open flame. Quite certainly he was burned, but he learned from this mistake: although fire was something beneficial, it was at the same time dangerous and had to be controlled if he hoped to benefit from its properties. Eating an unknown fruit was also risky; many were poisoned until the people could determine which fruits and vegetables were edible and safe. Later on, people learned that fruits that were bitten by birds were possibly edible. In the first stage, transmission of information was important to avoid repeating mistakes or risks, and thus early humans told their fellows not to eat certain fruits, not to approach predators, or to avoid certain high-risk locations. All this information was transmitted based on what was already known and likely included a detailed description of the dangerous animal or poisonous fruit. But when observers tried to tell their fellows of something that was totally out of the ordinary, the listeners did not accept it as easily. The narrator was then forced to say the events must have been the result of magic, and legends were born.

In the verification process that follows observation, we evaluate all possible causes and effects of the observed occurrence, provided, of course, that it can be compared to something already known. For example, the first human inhabitants realized that lightning bolts during a storm destroyed trees or animals; there was no doubt about the veracity of this. Similar repeated observations eventually were accepted as something possible that might occur again even if the causes were unknown. In the process of analysis, people involved also sought the causes, and this search for causes is how the sciences began. But man also realized that he was able to use or apply new knowledge even without full understanding of causes. An Indian in the jungle observed foreign explorers that multiple times produced flames by just pressing a button on a cigarette lighter. Having witnessed this, he had to acknowledge that it was possible and real.

The learning process involves the acceptance of any phenomena as real and possible and subject to a procedure by which another person could repeat it or observe its spontaneous repetition. It's like learning to drive a car: after we have seen others doing it, it's up to us to do the same. We can teach the Indian to produce flames at will by pressing the lighter even though he does not know that fuel and a spark are required to initiate the fire. Much of the progress of civilization is due to the use of processes and methods passed down from one generation to another without anyone knowing their causes, creating an empirical but transferable knowledge.

Throughout time the learning process turned ignorant laypersons into farmers, ranchers, craftsmen, artisans, and healers. Carrying out their jobs allowed them to repeat actions at will or apply acquired skills for practical purposes while ignoring the fundamentals of those actions. You can drive a car without knowing anything about motor mechanics; you can use a radio, telephone, or television without knowing anything about electronics. In such cases we are just users or operators. The implementation stage is independent of the causes and processes behind the effect. For example, a race car driver can be a champion even if he is a bad mechanic. Inversely a good mechanic can be a terrible driver. In any art, trade, or profession we can find bad, average, and excellent doers. According to their level of learning and mastery of the techniques, we use the terms *novice* or *apprentice*, as opposed to *professional* or *master*.

Because Qigong is an art or technical process that later became a science, it had to go, like the others, through all the stages listed above. Primitive Chinese peoples realized that their counterparts in certain circumstances did things they could not do under normal conditions. The primitive atmosphere was aggressive and inhospitable, and therefore humans were subject to many mishaps and natural disasters. Thus they observed that after an earthquake, someone desperate to rescue his family raised a large stone that exceeded normal forces. They also noted that a person who was chased by a beast jumped a distance that normally he would not have been able to accomplish in order to escape. They also observed the movements of the animals, whose sequences were the first replicated in ancient exercises of Qigong, known as Dao-yin. They also noticed that during festivals and dances people went into a kind of trance that allowed them to walk on burning coals and withstand other physical abuse without getting hurt. Healers who had learned the use of herbs by the knowledge transferred from generation to generation also realized that patients' conditions noticeably improved when the same healer mimicked a dance to "ward off evil spirits" and entered a trance that allowed him to exercise an unknown healing force on patients.

Our ancestors also noted that in certain circumstances they would have a hunch or intuitive feeling of a danger that threatened them, or they knew intuitively and inexplicably that a relative was in danger, which allowed them to go to that person's aid. All these abnormal events appear to have been a set of skills that some acknowledge as mechanisms for survival of the species and certainly were the basis of paranormal Qigong.

The verification stage, which follows replicating observed experiences, began when the healers in their ceremonies (including those to ward off spirits) realized that a procedure, when repeated, produced the same effect in almost all patients to whom it was applied. So it became a ritual, a public or private ceremony involving a programmed sequence of actions. That verification stage for paranormal Qigong was usually accomplished within the walls of monasteries, where monks had more time and chances to do trials. Their methods of meditation and mental concentration, which were used during the implementation phase, were improved, and the new information gathered was transmitted to novices by the experienced monks. Something similar happened with secular healers outside convents who transmitted information to their children or apprentices. These procedures, in principle available to many, were taken and improved by a reduced group of individuals, some of whom became best doers, obtaining fame, and got to be called masters. As time went on, the continuous observation and gathering of information on those unexplainable phenomena by ancient humans led them to determine that there was a "way to do" and that this way of doing, when repeated, produced the same results. They noticed as well that performers required a special state of mind, which at that time was achieved through rituals or ceremonies or, in some cases, by the ingestion of certain substances.

All of us, probably unknowing, exercise daily control over matter and energy at a first level that involves all physical and mental conscious processes of human beings, such as thinking, studying, walking, loving, eating, and sleeping. But there is a second level at which we can act in a different way because there we have access to physical and mental faculties that are considered unusual or extraordinary. This second or higher level is considered a state different from wakefulness or sleep; it is known by many names, such as higher state of consciousness, trance, ecstasy, samadhi, satori, fana, nirodha, contemplatio, kavvanah, hesykasm, and many others in each different language, religion, or culture. In modern science it is designated as an Altered (or Alternate) State of Consciousness, (ACS's)[49] and it is only during these ASCs that so-called miracles or wonders are accomplished.

During these altered states of consciousness, we can gain access to an unknown world where we can enhance our cognitive, intuitive, and parapsychic abilities; we can transmit and receive telepathic messages, capture the thinking of others, and enhance our physical capabilities to new levels of superpower or superstrength. In this state, the individual crosses the threshold from the conscious into the unconscious, whether individual or collective. Here the strength of intentionality is enhanced to unimagined limits to produce amazing and miraculous effects.

To voluntarily (not spontaneously) move from a normal state to an altered state of consciousness, requires a specialized method, one that serves only that purpose. That is the rule for many human activities that require a specialized procedure: even preparing a meal requires a recipe or instruction.

Any procedure or technique used to control subtle energy, Qigong included, implies risks for both the practitioner and the person who

---

49 See *Altered States of Consciousness* by Hilary Evans (Aquarian Press, 1989), *Altered States of Consciousness and Mental Health* by Colleen A. Ward (Sage Publications, 1989), and *Elemental Mind: Human Consciousness and the New Physics* by Nick Herbert (Plume, 1993).

receives the resulting action as a healing treatment. This differs from conventional medicine, in which the only one at risk is the patient. In martial arts applications, originally intended to develop a super strength for fighting in battles, the capabilities of superstrength and endurance were released in combat, but in normal daily life, warriors were just people like anyone else. Attempting to keep these enhanced capabilities all the time creates an imbalance with serious consequences because the energy is as bad in excess as it is in deficiency. Ancient texts and modern Qigong texts alike are full of warnings arising from the experience of our predecessors.

The Chinese, when referring to the balance necessary for sustaining life on this planet, refer to the theory of Yin and Yang. They noticed that problems were always produced by an imbalance. For instance, rain is good for crops, but excess rain creates floods that are destructive. By the same token, the lack of rain brings severe droughts that are also harmful and turn greenery into barren land. Many books written on this subject condense the knowledge as follows: something in excess is out of balance and should be on equal terms with its opposite. The Chinese elders found that the cosmos was orderly and harmonious and systematic as well. In this universe there was a union of opposites: heaven and earth, calm and movement, day and night, and so on.

The Chinese have a saying: "Spring and summer promote Yang; autumn and winter promote Yin." The Yang is the active, positive, or masculine part. In medicine Yang is linked to the properties of excess, hyperactivity, and overheating. Conversely, the Yin is the passive, female, or negative polarity. In medical terms, it is a deficiency.

All things have simultaneously a Yin and a Yang aspect. Take for example a mountain: its Yang side, toward the sun, is warm and bright while its Yin side has shade and is cold. The human body also has its Yin side, which is the trunk, the back, and the limbs, while the Yang side is the lower body, abdomen, and internal organs. The imbalance between Yin and Yang in the body produces disease. In modern medicine people are submitted to blood or urine tests to determine whether there is an imbalance of certain factors—a high cholesterol level, a low sugar level, and so forth. While initially *Yin* and *Yang* were used to describe only concrete things, with the development of human thought, they became abstract concepts as well. The Yang represents everything that is superficial, energetic, positive, upward, fast, intense, bright, open, distant, hot, and so on, while Yin is all that is innate, calm, slow, descending, dark, contractive, closed, and cold.

This ancient theory about the necessary existence of opposites has been confirmed at the subatomic level. In the early 1930s, British physicist Paul Dirac[50] predicted the existence of antiparticles: for every particle, there should be another fundamental atomic antiparticle with the same mass but with an electric charge in the opposite direction. Following the statement of this theory, it was verified in laboratories. Now we know that the antiparticle of an electron is a positron; of a proton, an antiproton; and of a quark (the most basic atomic particle), an antiquark.

The Yin and Yang are closely related to each other. In fact, one cannot exist without the other, although the two can be transformed by certain circumstances. They are entirely different in nature and restricted to one another. They are constantly changing, and the increase of one means the decrease of the other. It is through these incessant changes that things develop and life is maintained.

Qi as an energetic substance is also divided into *Yin qi*, which is heavy and tends to settle, and *Yang qi*, which is light and tends toward suspension. The purpose of Qigong practice is to establish an internal and external balance with the environment around us. Modern research and observation lead to the conclusion that the art or science of Qigong is based on two principles:

---

50 Paul Adrien Maurice Dirac (August 8, 1902–October 20, 1984) was an English theoretical physicist who made fundamental contributions to the early development of both quantum mechanics and quantum electrodynamics.

1. Control of subtle energy (qi) is an innate human ability that can be developed and increased just as humans can develop their physical abilities (athletes) or mental skills (scholars and researchers). Such a control capacity has been observed and reported in different cultures and historical times.

2. In order for one to access the controlling level (where exceptional activities can be performed) he or she must first access an altered state of consciousness. Such a scientifically defined state has many names, depending on the culture or religious movement where it has been reported.

However, simply accessing an altered state is not enough. What is important is that intentionality be released while one is in that state.

Notice that intentionality is not verbal (with words) like prayers. Intentionality at this level is the result of a previous conditioning process that allows this to be released in fractions of a second detached of any verbal procedure or thinking process. For instance, basic physics has taught us that it is necessary to apply force in order to move any object (mass or matter). What is not mentioned in traditional physics (because it is not its area of concern) is that even if we have the object (matter) and the energy or potential force to move it, it will not move if we do not complete the process by our conscious decision. Do we or don't we want to move it? This new (nonphysical) element is intentionality.

We could say that intention is not a concept in the exact sciences. True, it does not appear in any of the formulas we studied in physics and is not considered in relation to time, space, speed, and the like. But a revisionist physics should include intentionality as a coefficient in most of the formulas that exist in classical physics. Let's consider a simple example:

An object moving at a constant speed, say a car at forty miles per hour, after two hours will have traveled a distance calculated by the formula $d = v \times t$, in which d stands for distance (space), v stands for velocity (speed), and **t** stands for time. In our example **d** equals 40 × 2, or 80 miles.

But if the driver of the vehicle does not want it to move, he'll keep the brakes on, in which case intentionality would equal zero. And if he wants it to move, he'll step on the accelerator. Now intentionality equals one. Thus we can express intentionality by adding a coefficient to the formula, which we would call **I** = Intention, so the formula would be

$$\mathbf{d} = \mathbf{(I)}\ \mathbf{(v \times t)}.$$

If there is no intention, the coefficient is equal to zero, and the vehicle does not travel any distance, as zero as a multiplier will always produce a zero result. On the other hand, with positive intention, meaning a positive value (1) is used as a multiplier, the vehicle moves, and the traditional equation will yield normal results.

When we get out of classical (Newtonian) physics and enter the realm of quantum physics, intention is paramount. Remember when Schrödinger[51] established the cat paradox, by which a cat inside a closed box could be either alive or dead, so to verify which, the observer should open the box to see what's inside; only then does he really know whether the cat is alive or dead. It is the intention of the observer that "collapses the system" when transformed into action. For quantum physicists, the electron is not a particle revolving around the nucleus like planets in the solar system, an image used quite often to refer to atomic-related facts. For them, the electron is more like a cloud of possibilities about its possible location, and only by a measurement interaction would it be located in a certain place. Our life is full of possibilities. When we choose to do something or not do it, that action or lack of action changes the outcomes.

---

51   Erwin Alexander Schrödinger (August 12,1887–January 4, 1961) was an Austrian physicist who developed a number of fundamental results in the field of quantum theory, which formed the basis of wave mechanics. Schrödinger proposed an original interpretation of the physical meaning of the wave function and in subsequent years repeatedly criticized the conventional Copenhagen interpretation of quantum mechanics (using, for example, the paradox of Schrödinger's cat).

Intentionality is closely tied to desires. Either we want or don't want. Either we move or stop. Our convictions or moral values often modify our intentionality. That is, stopping to wonder whether a given course of action is good or appropriate causes us to hesitate. Intentions are the tools to change outcomes, although that is not always possible. Qigong helps people to enhance intentionally and facilitate outcomes that could be unexpected and sometimes considered miraculous. But nature imposes some limits that can never be surpassed, at least by humans.

If we go to a roulette table at a casino, we have the intention to win, and so we make bets on our preferred numbers. But we should be conscious that our intention to win will not necessarily be transformed into reality. One of the hindrances to our intentions (good or evil) is randomness, or chance—something that is imponderable, uncontrollable, and somewhat unpredictable. And although it is unpredictable, there are certain ranges within which a possibility could become a reality. This range is linked and somewhat offset by probability, which is the fact that something that in principle is possible could happen if certain conditions are present and that make it more or less likely. It is common to consider *probable* and *possible* as synonyms, but in the strict sense, they have different meanings. In physics it is demonstrated, for example, that it is always *possible* for electric discharges to produce lightning bolts, but their amount and frequency depend on the *probabilities*. If the weather is overcast with signs of a storm, it is *possible* and *probable* that there will be lightning bolts. On the other hand, the likelihood, or probability, is remote on a cloudless, sunny day: it is *possible* but not *probable*. The weather forecast is just a report that informs us about the low or high probabilities that it could rain, snow, and so forth. The general public is interested in those probabilities in order to take precautions. We all already know that it is always *possible* for a given weather condition to occur; we just do not know when. The important thing is *when* (probability), not *what* (possibility). If we play a lottery game, it is indeed possible that we could hit the jackpot, but it is not 100 percent probable: the odds could be one in several million. We know that in the sixties humankind reached the moon, and we all know that it is thus possible that any of us can go there, but it is unlikely—not probable—that you or I will do so. Sometimes when people do not obtain expected results, they say, "It is *probable* that I may not have done everything *possible*."

We are dealing with probability (the likelihood of an event) when we throw a coin and bet on which of the faces will be visible. The first two tosses may come up heads, the next tails, and so on. This is the product of chance or fortune, or, in more technical terms, these are random possibilities. But if we repeat the launch too many times, the odds will be reduced to 50 percent for each side because the coin has two sides only. If I throw a coin in the air many times and it almost always falls on the same side, this is against the odds. It likely means that a physical cause is interfering, like an imbalance in the material, or that an external agent has altered the odds. Qigong can be considered the external agent that changes outcomes, introducing an unbalance in the established mathematical probabilities.

CHAPTER 10

Altered States of Consciousness: The Access Gate

To enter most closed or restricted places (homes, offices, and so on) we need a key to unlock the front door. We also have passwords for our e-mail accounts and websites. In the case of controlling the vital subtle energy qi, we need to access a special level through a process that includes a change in our normal mental state. We require a method that could allow us to switch our mind to an altered (Alternate) state of consciousness. Gaining access to an altered state does not require an exclusive procedure; different methods and rituals have in fact been described in many cultures. However, in the past some persons surrounded those procedures with mystery and secrecy.

As this is an extensive and specialized topic, involving different areas of knowledge, like physiology, psychology, parapsychology, physics, and neurology, among others, I will make reference only to the main guidelines for the unacquainted reader. For a deeper analysis, I recommend a classic book on this subject, *Altered States of*

Consciousness by Charles T. Tart,[52] as well as another book that analyzes the topic deeply, *Altered States of Consciousness: A Book of Readings*[53]. The term *altered states of consciousness* was introduced in 1970 by the already mentioned Dr. Charles Tart, a psychologist at the University of California, Davis. Basically the origin and motivation of his work were the experiments with psychedelic drugs in vogue during the sixties. Tart insisted on new methods for the study of such phenomena, as the traditional and objective observer had no way to see inside the mind of a Yogi or any other person. He proposed that it was necessary to discard some objectivity and be a little more subjective to share the experience of the altered states because in such events the reality is relative, depending on the state of consciousness in which it is perceived.

Ronald K. Siegel, a psycho pharmacologist and the psychologist Hainrich Kluver of the University of Chicago observed similar patterns of altered states of consciousness on the experiences of subjects undergoing administration of psychedelic drugs and hallucinogenic substances like peyote mushrooms. They noticed that a recurring pattern existed in all these alterations of consciousness, and the descriptions of these states coincided with those reported by people with Parkinson's disease, heart attacks, central nervous system infections, and other neurological disorders. These patterns seemed also to occur in dreams or in people with severe migraine attacks. Not all altered-state experiences are necessarily associated with mental illnesses or influenced by drugs; it was observed that conditions such as deep meditative states or trance shared a pattern that enabled these to be included as altered states as well.

This new scientific term was aimed to include all anomalous states under investigation, which were considered outside the field of study

---

52   Charles T. Tart (born 1937) is an American psychologist and parapsychologist known for his psychological work on the nature of consciousness (particularly altered states of consciousness).

53   Charles T. Tart (author, editor), Arnold M. Ludwig (author), Arthur J. Deikman (author), Milton H. Erickson (author), Gerald Vogel (author), M. Bertini (author), David Foulkes (author), Frederik van Eeden (author), and Kilton Stewart (author).

of traditional science and had thus far been referred to by the term *metaphysics*, meant to encompass those events that were beyond the boundaries of known physical laws.

In our Western culture, one of the best-known versions of altered states is *ecstasy*. The term comes from Greek *ektasis*, which means "being out," and refers to a person's sense of being transported out of his or her routine of acting, feeling, and perception. Laski[54] describes three types of ecstasy: an *Adamic ecstasy*, which is perceived as a renewal and purification of the self, or ego, and accompanied by great happiness; *ecstasy of knowledge*, which includes a sense of revelation without direct contact with the source of knowledge; and a *knowledge-contact ecstasy*, which is often cited as a direct contact with the source of a so-called revelation, which could be a spirit, God, or an angel. This final type is what many consider to be a mystical experience.

Another well-known altered state of consciousness is the trance. The term *trance* derives from the Latin verb *transire*, which means "crossing" or "pass through." Traditionally it was thought that trance states were those in which the spirit momentarily went to the "beyond." The technique known as "Transcendental Meditation"®™ from Maharishi Maheshi Yoghi applies a similar concept in the sense that when entering the altered state of consciousness, one is said to "transcend." In contemporary literature, *trance* has a variety of meanings so that it has become something of a generic term, covering all altered states of consciousness. Pattison, Kahan, and Hurd[55] offer the following definition: "The state of trance is a form of consciousness in which the person although conscious, seems detached and insensitive to external and internal stimuli. These people act as if they were in their own world away from the immediate reality of their environment." Among the different types of trances described, the most common is the trance-dream or

---

54 Laski, M. *Ecstasy in Secular and Religious Experiences*. London: Cresset Press, 1961.

55 Pattison, E. M., Kahan, J., and Hurd, G. S. "Trance and Possesion States," B. B.Wolman and M. Ullman, eds., *Handbook of States of Consciousness*. New York: Van Nostrand Reinhold, 1986.

vision-type dream[56] that takes place while the individual is in an altered state of consciousness.

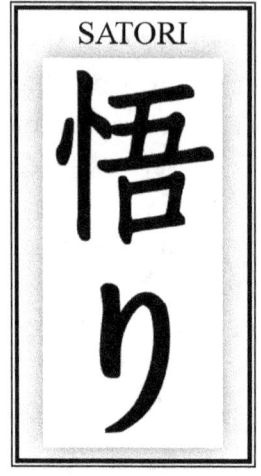

SATORI

Another name for the same phenomenon is *satori*, which comes from the Japanese verb *satoru* ("to know") and is the term used for awakening, comprehension, and understanding in Zen Buddhism. This experience is also referred *kenshō* ("seeing into one's true nature"). During this altered state, there is access to knowledge, and there is no distinction between the knower and the known (similar to *samyama* described in Patanjali's yoga). Satori is not the result of reasoning, since it requires a separation between thinking and the object of thought. This Japanese concept is very close to the idea of the altered state of consciousness, but it is charged with a Buddhist religious connotations.

The term *samadhi*, mentioned before, originally a Sanskrit word, also corresponds to an altered state. However, its exact definition is not so simple because it has several subtypes. In the *Bhagavad Gita*, there is a passage in which Arjuna asks Krishna about the signs evidencing that someone is in a state of samadhi. This is his reply:

> *When in your mind no desire is manifested, when you are not disturbed by any pain and not let yourself to be attracted by any pleasure, when you have no anger, no fear or passion... To access this state one should withdraw the senses from objects as a tortoise withdraws its head into the shell.*

Another term, *nirodha*, also from Sanskrit, is used to mean "cessation" or "destruction" and refers to an altered state of consciousness that

---

56 Read the book from the same author based on a vision-type dream: *Reincarnation and Hyperlink Theory* by Carlos J. Ruiz P. (2013).

can be accessed by those who have mastered the methods of Buddhist meditation. Literally it refers to the absence or extinction of a given entity. As the third of the four noble truths, it refers specifically to the cessation of *dukkha* and its causes; it is commonly used as a synonym for nirvana. It is the highest level in a sequence of states of mental concentration called *jhanas*. Buddhists use a method known as *Jhana meditation* to achieve a capability known as *shamatha*, or total calm. In this altered state of absolute calm, the meditator can practice *vipassana*, or introspective insight, to explore the nature of reality.

In the Catholic religion, the Latin term *contemplatio*, which can be translated as "contemplation," has been used since the early days of Christianity as a synonym for what today we know as meditation. At the beginning of the monastic tradition, when prayer formed part of the process of *lectio divina*, monks were subjected to four levels of religious discipline: *lectio, meditatio, oratio,* and *contemplatio. Lectio* was the reading of the scriptures, and *meditatio* (or *ruminatio*) was the reflection that followed the reading (at that time, the term *meditation* only referred to reflection and thorough analysis of an issue. *Oratio* was a prayer or deep thought, and finally *contemplatio* was the time after having surpassed the level of spoken communication and common thought at which point one entered an altered state. This contemplation was considered a mystical state—supernatural, infused, or extraordinary—and indicated that the intellect was operating in new way, one not brought about through effort. Beyond this fourth level was also a higher contemplation and, following it, mystical union. Saint Buenaventura (1221–1280) indicated three degrees in the contemplative process: the first exceeds the sensible world, in the second exceeds the intelligible, and in the third people seem to "enter a cloud."

In the Kabbalah, the masterpiece of Hebraic mysticism, the term *kavvanah* describes the altered state of consciousness. The common definition of *kavvanah* is "intention" or "concentration" during prayer or another ritual. Rabbis and Talmud scholars say that precise definition of this word has been elusive because it refers to an intangible inner state of mind, an abstract concept of thought, and not a physical or tangible action One method of concentration to enter this altered state was accessed through the repetition of alphabet letters (yud-heh-vav) [יהו] as a mantra. *Sefer Yetzirah* (*The Book of Creation*)[57] lists thirty-two different states of consciousness. The same book makes a distinction between two states of mind: "One can only visualize the *Sephiroth* in the consciousness state of *Chokhmah* (Wisdom) which is the nonverbal state of the mind (transcendent state)", and adds that such a state is very difficult to maintain. It is associated with the power of intuitive insight, flash-lightning like across consciousness. It is said that only in this altered state do prophecies occur.

The Sufis, who are mostly an esoteric branch of Islam, although originally there were also Christian Sufis (Masihi-i-Batini) call the state of meditation *muraqaba*. They use the term *fanaa* to define the altered state in which people lose their own identity; whose Arabic translation would be "annihilation" or "cessation." Sufis describe three stages in the meditation process, the first called *ghanood*; the second, *adraak*; and the third, *warood*. This third stage starts when mental concentration is sustained and somnolence is at a minimum. As soon as the mind is focused, the spiritual eye is activated. The conscious mind is not used to see through the spiritual eye, so concentration comes and goes. Gradually, the mind gets used to this kind of vision, and mental focus is sustained. With practice, the visions become so deep that the person starts considering himself a part of the experience rather than considering himself an observer. (This effect is similar to the *samiama* in the *Yoga Sutras*). To achieve this state, Sufis undergo intense study and practice, including the removal of bad inclinations (*an-nafs al-ammarah*) and feelings of guilt (*an-nafs al-lawwamah*).

Continuing with our comparison, in the ancient Orthodox Christian Church, the term *hesykasm* (from *hesychia* in Greek, which means "inner silence") was used extensively to refer to the altered state that was

---

57 Sefer Yetzirah: *The Book of Creation in Theory and Practice* by Aryeh Kaplan Ed. Samuel Weiser Inc. York Beach Maine.

achieved by constant repetition (like a mantra) of the words *kyrie eleison*, which is the short form in Greek for "Lord, have mercy on us." Saint John of Sinai commented that Hesykasm is the enclosing of the bodiless primary Cognitive faculty of the soul in the body. Any ecstatic states or other unusual phenomena that may occur in the course of such practice are considered secondary and unimportant, even quite dangerous. A special bodily position and the practice of breathing rhythmically while invoking a divine name seem to be common to both Jewish Merkabah mysticism and Christian Hesykasm. Thus the practice may have origins in the ascetical practices of the biblical prophets.

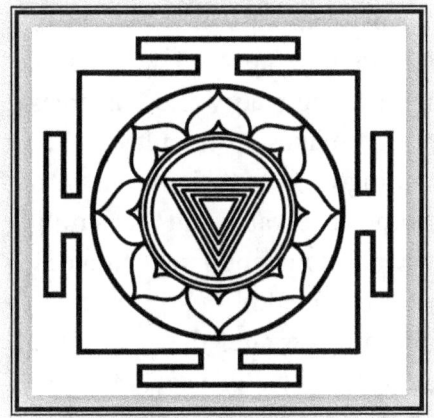

In Tibet, Buddhist groups called *Manggyapa* have among their rituals to gain access to an altered state of consciousness a prolonged and fixed observation of drawings known as mandalas or yantras. These are abstract geometrical figures or mystic diagrams engraved on a plaque usually made out of silver or copper. They are also drawn on parchment, skin, or special paper, using various colors and following an ancient method of preparation. Sometimes they are made using colored sand. As a tool for meditation employed by Tibetan monks, these yantras are combined with visualization techniques to transcend to higher states of consciousness. The yantra or mandala has no intrinsic power, but it aids in the deep concentration necessary to access altered states of consciousness.

The preceding information, which is neither complete nor limited, reveals that the concept of altered states of consciousness has been known and used in many different cultures and environments since remote times. It is not anything new. Though the names for it might be different, the characteristics are strikingly similar. In simple terms the altered state of consciousness can be compared to those reverie states in which daydream is the threshold between sleep and waking, either when we are falling asleep or when we are about to wake up. It would be the interpolation between being fully awake (when brain waves, measured with an EEG, show a predominance of beta rhythms, (from 13–30Hz)[58] and being sound asleep (when delta waves, less than 4 Hz, predominate). In the altered state of consciousness accessed in deeper states of meditation, trance, or hypnosis, there is a predominance of alpha waves (8–13 Hz) combined with theta waves (4–8 Hz). Let's remember that these measurements are collateral effects that in some way reflect the inner state of being in an altered state, somewhat like deducting which team is winning just by hearing the shouting from outside the stadium.

In altered states, whether induced or spontaneous, individual suffer to some extent an isolation from the surrounding reality and a decrease in the concept of their personal identity that makes it difficult for them to be detached from any of the surrounding objects ("Union with the One," as the mystics say). There are also some observable and measurable physiological effects, like a decrease of the basal metabolism, changes in heart rate, and alteration in breathing patterns. In addition, the electrical resistance of the skin changes, and the brain waves alter their pattern of predominance. Inhibition is reduced, and referral patterns over time are altered as well (known as time warp). These physiological changes have been clearly identified in laboratories in Qigong masters, Yogis, or people with enhanced extrasensory perceptions. A.M. Ludwig [59] mentions ten characteristics of altered states of consciousness: (1) changes in thinking, including extraordinary ideas about causes and effects, (2) loss or distorted sense of time, (3) loss of control over some voluntary functions of the body, (4) extreme emotions, ranging from panic to bliss, (5) body image distortions and disappearance of boundary between the self and

---

58 This is measured with an electroencephalogram (EEG), which is a testing machine that measures and records the electrical activity of the brain. Special sensors (electrodes) are attached to the head and hooked by wires to a computer. The computer records the brain's electrical activity on the screen or on paper as wavy lines.

59 Ludwig, A. M. *Altered States of Consciousness.* In "Trance & Possessive States." R Prince. Ed. Montreal: R.M. Bucke Memorial Society, 1968.

the collective, (6) perceptual disturbances, including hallucinations, delusions, and synesthesia, (7) changes in the meaning of things, including feelings of deep introspection and revelation, (8) a sense that the experience cannot be described in words or perhaps remembered, (9) feelings of rejuvenation or rebirth, and (10) increased suggestibility. As we can see, the interaction of mind over matter and energy makes the latter pass into the background.

It is curious to note that in ancient times three mental states were described in India as follows: waking, sleeping, and dreaming. In the West, on the other hand, until a few decades ago, only two states were accepted—waking and sleeping. Later that division disappeared when REM sleep was observed, a state of sleep during which a fast circular movement of the eyeballs occurs. These movements clearly determined that the dream state (whether the dreams were pleasant or nightmares) was different from sleep, which thus defined a third state. But the Vedic literature of India identifies a fourth state of consciousness, one that is different from the other three known in Indian culture. This fourth state, called *turiya*[60], is also known as "the superconscious state," which is basically the equivalent of our modern altered state of consciousness. The state of *turiya*, which is the Sanskrit term for the "fourth," was seen as an important clue about the nature of consciousness. It is said that the induced state of *turiya* is similar to the spontaneous state known as *anandamaya*. Verse VII of the Mandukya Upanishad[61] describes this fourth state as follows:

---

60 In Hindu philosophy, *turiya* (caturiya, chaturtha) is the experience of pure consciousness. It is the background that underlies and transcends the three common states of consciousness (waking consciousness, dreaming, and dreamless sleep). See *Alternative Realities, the Paranormal, the Mystic, and the Transcendent in Human Experience* by Leonard George, (Facts on File Inc., New York, 1995, p.283).

61 The Mandukya Upanishad is the shortest of the Upanishads, the scriptures of Hindu Vedanta. It is in prose, consisting of twelve verses expounding the mystic syllable *aum*; the three psychological states of waking, dreaming, and sleeping; and the transcendent fourth state of illumination.

> *Turiya neither inward-turned nor outward-turned consciousness, nor the two together; not an undifferentiated mass of consciousness; neither knowing, nor unknowing; invisible, ineffable, intangible, devoid of characteristics, inconceivable, indefinable, its sole essence being the consciousness of its own Self; the coming to rest of all relative existence; utterly quiet, peaceful, blissful, without a second: this is the Ātman, the Self, this is to be realized.*

Our intention so far, is to make it clear that paranormal phenomena always occur under altered states of consciousness, and Qigong is no exception. Its training practices require access to an altered state, but without the aid of psychedelic drugs, rituals, or conditioning procedures (visual or sonic). Qigong masters have the great advantage of being able to transition from a normal waking state to an altered state without resorting to any outside assistance, and they are even able to do so without attracting the notice of anyone around them.

Unlike other procedures and rituals, such as the dances of the dervishes (Islamic Sufis), the beating drums in ceremonies of Brazilian Macomb, and Tibetan mental concentration with aid of mandalas, the practice of Qigong neither creates nor requires any previous mental conditioning that would make access to the altered state difficult, slow, or complicated. Other procedures become something like the conditioned reflex in the experiment of Pavlov's dogs. All of them pursue the same objective, but they vary in their external methods. Followers of different methods usually affirm that their method is the best; often they omit making reference to other methods because that would reduce the value of their own. The desire of a few to control and dominate many others causes them to publicize an overvalued idea of their own rituals, disregarding the final purpose. For them it seems the road is more important than the destination. Unfortunately many of the methods or procedures to access an altered state of consciousness were initially offered as rituals within a dogmatic, religious, or exclusive environment.

For that reason many people have mistaken the means with the purpose, especially if there were interests that induced them to believe so.

In the past, in those communities and societies physically and culturally isolated from their surroundings, people assumed their rituals were true and valuable and the only method to access altered states of consciousness. Along with knowledge of the rituals, this attitude was transmitted from one generation to the next. Thus people adopted those rituals that were dominated by a small, exclusive group of leaders who in this way were able to have power and control over others.

I strongly believe that Qigong procedures are a human inheritance that should be shared by all. Today, in a world already considered a global village, we have realized that all human beings have similar inborn capacities and are therefore able to perform the same actions. We are lucky to benefit from a sub product of cultural globalization, which is the information we receive from many other cultures. And often we find that we are using different methods or approaches as those in other cultures to get to the same outcome. There are no variations in the final results and their applications, whether those achieved by the Qigong masters in China or obtained by the Yogis in India, and in general, for those obtained in cultures that intuitively make or have made use of the outcomes while controlling vital energy (qi). For some of us Qigong has two advantages: its detachment from rites and the fact that it is subject of study and research by scientific and academic institutions.

In contemporary studies researchers have concluded that altered states of consciousness can be of three different types. The first is spontaneous. These are involuntary, not induced, and can be activated or triggered by several causes. The second is induced, but not voluntary nor provoked. It is typically a consequence of diseases or environmental factors. The third is induced specifically by procedures or rituals of various kinds or by administration of psychedelic drugs.

Among the spontaneous states, the first type, we can mention the prophetic dreams, visions or premonitions, lucid dreams, experiences during sleep known as astral travel, the sleep paralysis that occurs when a person is awake and conscious but unable to move, sleepwalking, hypnotic effects produced by traveling some very straight roads, and so forth. There are also spontaneous altered states associated with specific cultures, such as pibloktoq, which often occurs among Eskimo women. During these events, these women tear off their clothes and jump into near-freezing water, where they can swim and remain without suffering. Sometimes they also crawl naked and act like dogs, barking and rolling in the snow without feeling the freezing cold.

The second group of altered states, which are externally but not intentionally induced, are those caused by physical illnesses such as hysteria, amnesia, some forms of sleepwalking, dissociation of personality, and the like. Such states could also be induced by environmental effects, such as severe deprivation of food, prolonged enclosure or confinement, sensory deprivation, and as well by changes in body chemistry, body electricity, fatigue or exhaustion, injury or pain, imminent danger of death, and so on.

Finally, we have the third kind, which are externally and purposely induced, either through certain rituals or by experimental procedures in laboratories of research institutions. Among the experimentally induced procedures can be mentioned the use of stroboscopic flashes of light (photic stimulation) and sounds of different types, like drums, bells, or rattles (sonic stimulation). In this category we can include as well the so-called biofeedback procedure that uses electronic devices and instruments to condition the brain to react under certain stimuli. Some of these devices include special lenses and headphones to induce altered states, but according to some researchers, the use of these devices outside the labs is not advisable, as they could damage the cerebral cortex.

To complete the list of externally induced altered states, we should mention the chemically induced procedures, most of which include the use of hallucinogenic, psychotropic, or psychedelic substances, either from natural sources or synthetic drugs. In ancient times during religious rituals, people used to smear the body with ointments containing sundew.[62] The ointments produced altered states when the skin absorbed the plant compounds. Also in this group of chemically induced altered states are those brought on by the ingestion of hallucinogenic mushrooms that contain the psychotropic tryptamines psilocybin and psilocin (some species also contain weaker psychotropic compounds like baeocystin or norbaeocystin). The *peyote* cactus (*Lophophora williamsii*) is also a plant used to produce altered states due to its content of mescaline. It is said that Native Americans are likely to have used peyote for at least 5,500 years. There are hundreds of plants with varying hallucinogenic effects, like the *ayahuasca* in Peru. Among the drugs made in laboratories, the most common are LSD, DMT, mescaline, and DOB.

Smoking certain substances, such as hashish or marijuana, can also induce an altered state. In the past burning incense was used in Catholic religious ceremonies. This induced mild altered states that people associated with a pleasant environment, which motivated them to return often to enjoy that pleasurable feeling.

To make a list of all the things that may induce an altered state of consciousness is almost impossible. According to anthropologist Rob Shultheiss,[63] the following unusual actions can induce an altered state: "smoke three pipes of strong tobacco after two days of fasting," "pedal an exercise bike in a dark room for five hours," or "keep watching the signal pattern that some television stations broadcast while out of the air until dawn" (those look like a Tibetan mandala).

Basically, all the procedures used to enter an altered state require a high degree of concentration and detachment from the external environment. These high levels of concentration are perfectly described in the system of raja-yoga and *Yoga Sutras* of Patanjali:

The first level begins with a simple "scattered attention," similar to our attention when we walk down a street and observe buildings, vehicles,

---

62 Also known as drosera, these sundews comprise one of the largest genera of carnivorous plants, with at least 194 species.

63 See "Secrets of the Inner Mind: A Journey through the Mind and Body," chapter 3 (p. 74) in *Altered States*, Time-Life Books, Richmond, VA.

and pedestrians simultaneously. Our attention is divided between the road and the background environment. In that moment we are aware that there are vehicles moving and other people within our walking perimeter.

But when something that arouses our attention enters into our field of vision, whether an acquaintance or a vehicle sounding its horn, our vision focuses for a short time on that person or action in order to determine what it is or where it comes from. This attention, almost subconscious, is basically an early defense mechanism that persists in modern humans. (In primitive conditions, humans did not know if the image or sound approaching was a predator or represented a risk.)

Once our brain discriminates what kind of object or person is within our field of view, it usually returns quickly and quietly to its routine, unless the person or object has something peculiar, in which case the object or person holds our attention, replacing or superseding attention to our previous activity. In this case our attention now is focused on the new person or object, and what surrounds us is no longer important. Therefore we say that there was something that "caught our attention." Moving to this focused attention provides access to the second level.

That second level of focused attention occurs when someone carefully observes a sculpture in a museum or when a collector takes an object to identify it. In such circumstances the individual's surroundings fade to the background while he or she carefully observes and scrutinizes every detail of an object. When the focusing is passive, for instance when we are the object of observation, there occurs a paranormal phenomenon by which we can sense that someone is watching us intently. This is called "the sense of being stared at[64]."

The third level is the deepest, and it involves "complete abstraction" or total detachment from one's surroundings. Concentration is focused solely on what is being done, and time passes without one's realizing

---

64 See *The Sense of Being Stared At, and Other Aspects of the Extended Mind* (2003) by Rupert Sheldrake (Inner Traditions, Rochester, VT) and, in *Journal of Consciousness Studies* (Vol. 12, No. 6, 2005), "Sheldrake and His Critics: The Sense of Being Glared At."

it. A portraitist inspired while painting or a musician composing a melody is at that level. This not only happens to artists, who in ancient times were said to be inspired by a muse[65], but to ordinary beings, too, when they are profoundly focused on their work. This might include an engineer developing a drawing, a researcher looking for something under a microscope, or an accountant squaring a balance. There now exists extensive literature that investigates that phenomenon of high concentration, called *flowing*[66]. Researchers found that mental, athletic, or artistic performances are super enhanced in this state and observed physiological reactions as well, such as changes in oxygen consumption, heart palpitations, altered metabolism, decreased levels of sensory skin, and others.

These same three levels of ordinary thought have an equivalent gradation in meditative (or contemplative) abstract thinking. If we sit at rest in a chair in a quiet place, perhaps with very faint light or total lack of it, we can concentrate our abstract thoughts on some object or person. In fact, when we are in love or have a serious problem, our thoughts easily focus on the person or problem.

To summarizing, these different levels are well described in the *Yoga Sutras* of Patanjali. At the first level we focus our thoughts on an object or person (this level is called *dharana*). At the second level our focus intensifies, and everything around us seems to disappear (this level is called *dhyana*). The third level of concentration is the most difficult to achieve. At this level the observer is in a state of total abstraction (called *samadhi*), and the observer and observed object are nearly fused. But the important thing is that only while immersed in the third level are we

---

65 The term refers to an imaginary being, person, or force that gives someone ideas and helps the individual to write, paint, or make music. It is a concept that originated in Greek and Roman mythology, comprising each of nine goddesses, the daughters of Zeus and Mnemosyne, who preside over the arts and sciences.

66 Flow is the mental state of operation in which a person performing an activity is fully immersed in a feeling of energized focus, full involvement, and enjoyment in the process of the activity. In essence, flow is characterized by complete absorption in what one does. This term was introduced by Mihály Csíkszentmihályi.

able to maximize our intentionality, increase our physical powers, and capture, move, and emit subtle energy. But reaching that level is not easy!

Many mystical or esoteric movements linked to religions have used their rituals to access the altered states of consciousness and their associated phenomena as a means of seizing and proselytizing new adherents. Undoubtedly this is a direct consequence of the ignorance of people who are unaware that the preparatory ritual is not the most important aspect or that the ritual in question is not the only means to accessing an altered state. The ancient Romans had a saying, "All roads lead to Rome," which could be applied in another context. There are different ways to gain access to that special mental state required to control qi. Elaborate rituals are not required, nor are rules or codes of submission that are often imposed on adherents of various groups. For meditation alone, there are at least fifty-two different methods described in the specialized literature.

In the recent past, some people intended to cover the sun with one finger and simply denied the veracity of a series of unexplained phenomena, leaving them outside rigorous scientific scrutiny. But advances made in the fields of parapsychology, biology, and neuroscience (which at first were intended only to accumulate the evidence of a series of cases in a regular and systematic way) produced undeniable results. Statistically speaking, the bulk of evidence accumulated surpassed the mathematical probabilities (odds ratio) that these cases could be due to randomness, and this forced researchers to start the pursuit for the causes that influenced the statistical data.

For those who sometimes forget what the mathematical odds ratio[67]is, I remind them that in simple terms it is a reference number to compare the ratio of the probability of an event's occurring to the probability of its not occurring. Or you can think of it as the chances or likelihood of success of existing possibilities.

---

67 An odds ratio (OR) is a measure of association between an exposure and an outcome. The OR represents the odds that an outcome will occur given a particular exposure compared to the odds of the outcome occurring in the absence of that exposure.

One way to verify that actually a system can be influenced, and that experimental results could be changed, is when we manage to repeat a phenomenon a number of times exceeding the odds ratio. This method is the most commonly used in testing extrasensory phenomena, about which we are still largely unaware of the causes behind the changes. But fortunately we can measure the results and see if they are outside the range of fortuitous chance and rate of probabilities. This is an integral part of any scientific researching method.

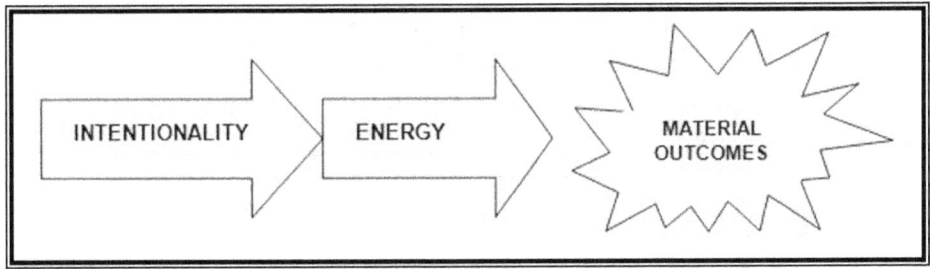

History is full of examples of how the intentionality manifested during an altered state of consciousness induces changes in outcomes at unexpected levels. Proof of this is that in all the training that mystics undergo, there is a common factor—the renouncing of desires. This seems to be a paradox: on the one side, they are trained to do many things we all want, but on the other, they give most of them up. That suppression of desires has a logical foundation. Although the person is able to accomplish many things, he doesn't know if these desires, when met, will produce the intended benefits or be returned as a boomerang against him. It is difficult to limit how far and where rational desire starts to become a whim. The ancients said that the worst thing that could happen to a person is that all his wishes would be met, and a clear example is the ancient Greek myth of King Midas, who wished that everything he touched would become gold so that he would be the richest in the world. Eventually he died of starvation because, as he'd wished, any food he touched became gold.

CHAPTER 11

Who is in the Cockpit: Is It the Mind, the Psyche, or the Spirit?

There is a continuous and endless debate over which part of our human system is in control, which part transforms our intentions into actions the way a pilot does when deciding when to land or take off.

For ancient humans existence was simple. According to them, we have a material component, our body, and a nonmaterial one. They arrived at this simple conclusion after realizing that thoughts, emotions, and affections were not material. They could not grasp love, hate, and the like.

The ancient Greeks discriminated the *psyche* (immaterial) and the *physis* (material). In more ancient writings from China and India, not only is the separation between the material and nonmaterial mentioned, but they also began to speak of a third energy component—qi or prana, respectively. This third component later was known in the West as the vital force or élan vital, and this concept initiated a doctrine known as vitalism[68]. This affirms that living organisms are fundamentally different from nonliving entities because they contain some nonphysical element

---

68 See: Bechtel, William and Robert C. Richardson (1998). Vitalism. In E. Craig (Ed.), Routledge Encyclopedia of Philosophy. London: Routledge.

or are governed by different principles than those of the inanimate things.

Our predecessors realized that their physical bodies were attached to an invisible force or energy that kept them alive and active. They thought it was the air because when people stopped breathing, they died. They also noticed that their physical energy would fluctuate: sometimes they felt strong and active, and at another times they felt weak and vulnerable. And regardless of their physical capacity, their thoughts and feelings seemed to act independently. For this reason they started defining two immaterial elements linked to our bodies; hence the concepts of soul and spirit were introduced. *Soul* was a synonym for vitality or energy, and *spirit* was a synonym for mind or psyche. Due to translation errors likely brought about by religious interests (or, in other cases, by ignorance) these two separate elements were taken as synonymous, and religions started talking about a single element, the soul, even though there were two different concepts. Nevertheless the two different words persisted in time and were used in dissimilar contexts. As Qigong is based on manipulation of vital energy by a control element, it is important to make it clear what these two immaterial components really are.

Applying some basic physics, we realize that we are a human system. This system is based on the interaction of various components whose number has been under scientific and philosophical debate for a long time and continues to be so to this day. In this debate are included logical and very scientific arguments, but it seems that these arguments clash not only with certain preconceived religious dogmas but also with profitable interests associated with power and domination.

In our modern conception, the most logical division of the human system is into three separate components: matter (the body), energy (the soul), and a control element (mind or spirit). Understanding as energy (soul) the force that generates and maintain life in our organism. In the past some explained this division by making a comparison to objects or events in our daily lives, such as a vessel (material object) that was moved by the wind (energy) and was steered by a helmsman (control element).

Without wind (energy) the vessel could not sail; with wind but without control, the ship sails adrift and get lost. Only through a combination of the three elements could an effective action be achieved. We can now give many other similar examples, in which the material object (car, train, ship, or plane) is powered by a fuel (energy) and must have a driver or captain to lead (control element). Any industrial machinery has the same features: the object (the machine), energy (electricity or fuel), and someone to operate it (control element).

A friend of mine who is a mechanical engineer always elucidates philosophical problems from the point of view of building something, and he provided an additional example to clarify the role of the control element: "Tell me," he said, "what is the difference between these objects, all three made out of steel—a cooking pot, a tool, and a sword?" And then he added, "All of them require the same raw material, and, all three also require energy and labor, but what really makes them different is the design, plan, or instructions to produce each. So it is indeed the control element that determines the difference, for the material and energy could be the same."

The debate among theologians and philosophers was initiated a long time ago, and they were divided: some claimed that man was composed of two parts, body and soul, while others argued a threefold nature—body, soul, and spirit. Many like me refer to this latter conception as a Trichotomy. It is now known in English-speaking countries as the SSB Group (Spirit, Soul, and Body). This return to the awareness of the existence of three parts, not two, as has been taught by Christianity

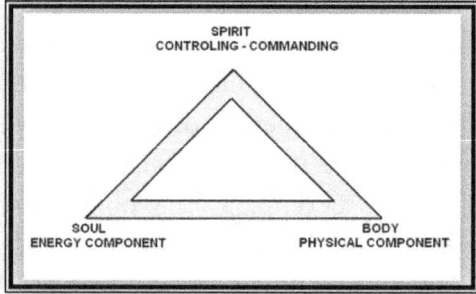

over the centuries, is a proof that formerly people had a clearer understanding of the human being, which now is taken up, strengthened, and renewed by the investigations of the sciences.

To accurately and fully define the concepts of soul (as energy component) and spirit (as a control element) is quite complicated. The first problem is that there is much confusion in the speakers of our language, not only because of the multiple meanings given to words, but because of the individual religion or belief system of each speaker. The second problem is the use of words that take on a different meaning when used in popular discourse and the translation of words or meanings from cultures with different values or knowledge. For our purposes it is necessary to make a clear distinction between the control component and the energy component because the first acts on the second to affect a third party.

Scholars and theologians (and this is not a religious discussion) argue that the current difference between the Christian Bible[69] and Jewish scriptures comes from mistranslations from Hebrew into Greek, then from Greek into Latin, and finally into some Romance languages. In the first translation into Greek, the words took on a connotation that was not the author's original Hebrew meaning, promoting ideas and concepts foreign to the Jewish mind. Later Greek translations into Latin were mostly accomplished by Christian monks in cloistered convents, and the way they perceived the world and their medieval ideas influenced the translators. For terms that were unclear, they sought similarities with something familiar and already known to them.

When we read the translations of these writings, we note that despite misinterpretations and errors, sometimes they indeed established a difference when using *soul* and *spirit*. Regarding the concept of soul in both biblical languages, *nefesh* (Hebrew) and *psyche* (Greek), though applied to an immaterial component, it was closely linked to the human body as part of it. The spirit, on the other hand, *ruach* (Hebrew) and *pneuma* (Greek) was accepted as something nonmaterial, but it could be separated and independent of the human body. This is demonstrated by the existence of "free spirits," alien and nonhuman,

---

69 Different religious groups include different books in their biblical canons, in varying orders, and sometimes divide or combine books or incorporate additional material into canonical books. Christian Bibles range from the sixty-six books of the Protestant canon to the eighty-one books of the Ethiopian Orthodox.

such as angels, archangels, seraphim, cherubim, ghosts, and demons. And in monotheistic Abrahamic religions such as Christianity, Judaism, and Islam it is generally accepted that these free spirits have controlling and interacting capacities in the material realm. The Jewish scriptures differentiate spirit (ruach) from mind or intellect (*neshamah*), and they consider three immaterial parts in the human system, *ruach, nefesh* and *neshamah, that would be equivalent to soul, spirit and mind (intellect).*

Ancient Hebrew Scriptures used up to five terms to express incorporeal levels: nefesh (soul), ruach (spirit), neshamah (intellect), chayah (vitality), and yechidah (uniqueness). Of these five, only the first three, nefesh, ruach, and neshamah, are considered to be part of the human being, while yechidah and chayah are considered wraps (*makifin*).

Christian scriptures began to handle the concept of spirit from the Book of Creation, Genesis, where it is said that life was insufflated into man as a breath (*ruach* in Hebrew). For those people, the difference between being alive or dead was determined by breathing, so it made sense that life was started like a breath. From that idea comes the phrase used when a person dies: people say "expired" or "gave her last breath." In the New Testament, the theologians say that the word *spirit* suffered additional meanings and connotations as influence from the Greco-Roman world and some Zoroastrians and Persians.

It seems that certain concepts were already quite clear to some Christians, like Saint Paul; it was he who said that the man was a trinity like his creator and so possessed a physical body, a soul, and a spirit. In the First Epistle of Saint Paul to the Thessalonians (1, 5:23) he said, "And the very God of peace sanctify you wholly, and may your whole *spirit and soul and body* be preserved blameless unto the coming of our Lord Jesus Christ" (italics mine). In Hebrews 4:12, it is written, "For the word of God is living and active, sharper than any two-edged sword, piercing and cutting *the soul and spirit*, joints and marrow and discerning the thoughts and intentions of the heart." (italics mine). These biblical references are cited not as a dogma but as a reference to a historical narrative showing that formerly there was a trichotomy[70], a concept that was then mistakenly—or intentionally—transformed into a dichotomy.

In the Islam faith, the holy Qur'an and Sunnah give us only a limited knowledge concerning the soul. From it we can say that the Arabic words *ruh* and *nafs* are both used, sometimes interchangeably, for the soul. (This is similar to the ambiguities in the Christian religion). For them *ruh* is an entity that differs entirely from the physical body (is immaterial). They coincide with the Jews when they say that the life was insufflated into the body as a breath (*ruach* for Jews and *ruh* for Islam). Scholars say that there is some difference in the way the words *ruh* and *nafs* are used. *Ruh* is the subtle spirit that resides in the heavens and needs a physical body to carry it on the earth. When this spirit is given a body, life begins, and soul is described as *nafs* (equivalent to the Hebrew *nephesh*). The word *nafs* is used in a number of ways in the Qur'an, all of which imply the meaning of a soul in a body. To my understanding, *ruh* is the free spirit, making *nafs* the live-force (soul). Following Aristotle, the Muslim philosophers Avicenna (Ibn Sina) and Ibn al-Nafis further elaborated on the Aristotelian understanding of the soul and developed their own theories. They both made a distinction between the soul and the spirit, and, in particular, the Avicennian doctrine on the nature of the soul was influential among the Scholastics.

The Chinese, especially the Taoists, have always believed in the existence of three main components of the human system: (1) substance or matter (*ching*), (2) energy (*qi* 气), which has two variations—*hun* and *po*[71]—and is equivalent to soul, and (3) spirit (*shen* or *ling-shen* 精神). Chinese medicine considers *shen* to be one of the "three treasures" that constitute life: *jing*, the essence; *qi*, the life-force; and *shen*, the spirit. Some add the mind (*yi*) as a subcomponent linked to the body. An

---

70 The philosophical idea that human nature consists of three parts,—body, soul, and spirit— is designated by the term *trichotomy*. The tripartite conception of humans originated in Greek philosophy, which conceived of the relation of the body and the spirit of humans to each other after the analogy of the mutual relation between the material universe and God.

71 Hun (魂) expresses the idea of continuous propagation, unresting flight; it is the qi of the lesser yang, working in man in an external direction, and it governs the nature or the instincts. Po (魄) expresses the idea of a continuous pressing urge on man; it is the qi of the lesser yin, and works in him, governing the emotions.

old adage from Qigong masters recommends to those who are new to the practice, "Yuh shen yii chi," which means to use the spirit (*shen*) to master the energy (*qi*). (In our Western culture, it would be something like saying to use the spirit to control the soul). In Taoism one's soul or energy is considered to be interlocked with the vital energy, which is what nourishes the soul. Ridding the body of impurities can increase this energy. The concept of soul in Shintoism (the native Japanese religion) is fairly vague. The word *tama* is used, which means "beautiful jewel" or "mysterious rock," to describe a soul. A variation of this is *tamashii*, which means "ball wind" (this would correlate it with the ancient words for spirit in other languages, suggesting air or breath). Even cultures that we consider a bit primitive, such as Haitian voodoo, distinguish four components, one material (*corps cadaver*), and three nonmaterial: *gros bon ange/gwo bonanj* (energy, soul, life-force, invisible core, vital spirit), petite bon ange or *ti bonanj* (consciousness or mind), and mét-tét (the spirit inhabitant the body, one of the Iwa).

Ancient Egyptians already considered a difference between the *Ba* (an insubstantial part of the personality often translated as "spirit") and the *Ka*, the soul. In the Sankhya school of philosophy from India, the spirit (*purusha*) is different from the soul (*jiva* or *atman*), and both are distinct from matter (*prakrti*). Other schools of India say that the name of soul is just a label for a set of constituents that are like wrappers, some thick and others more subtle (a similar concept to *makifin* of the Jewish scriptures).

I do not think that it is the product of chance or coincidence that in many languages there are two different words (*soul* and *spirit*) to refer to nonmaterial parts of our human system. So why does this difference exist? The spirit comes from the Latin word *espiritus* and is mentioned in the Christian Bible more than five hundred times. This etymological difference between the energy (soul) and the spirit has remained in many languages: in Spanish, *alma* (soul) and *espiritu* (spirit); in German, *Seele* (soul) and *Geist* (spirit); in French, *âme* (soul) and *esprit* (spirit); in Italian, *anima* (soul) and *spirito* (spirit); in Portuguese, *alma* (soul) and *espírito* (spirit); in Russian ДУХ (spirit) and ДУША (soul).

104

Trichotomy Concepts around the World

In Languages

English	body	soul	spirit	mind
Spanish	cuerpo	alma	espiritu	mente
French	corps	âme	esprit	esprit
German	Körper	Seele	Geist	Geist
Italian	corpo	anima	spirito	mente
Portuguese	corpo	alma	espírito	mente
Russian	тело	ДУША	ДУХ	ум/разум
Chinese	人体 Ren ti	灵魂 Ling hun	精神 Jing shen	心神 Yi
Hebrew	ףנ Guf	המש Nephesh	חַ Ruach	Neshamah

In Religions and Philosophy

Early Christians	Body	Soul	Spirit	
Jewish	Guf ףנ	Nephesh המש	Ruach חַ	Neshamah
Islam		Nafs	Al-Ruh	
Ancient Greeks	Soma	Psyche	Pneuma	
India - Sankhya School		Jiva and/or Atman	Purusha	Mana
Early Egyptians	Khat	Ka	Ba	
Japanese Sintoist		Tama	Tama-shii	

Who introduced the confusion between these terms that were so clearly differentiated in the past? Why should we have to remove so much dust from old books to find again these ancient truths? When was it that people started to confuse the spirit with the soul?

The preceding comments on the trichotomy concept have the only purpose of demonstrating that different immaterial components of the human systems seem to have been accepted in many cultures. In fact it is quite irrelevant what ancients though about these components since their scientific knowledge at that time was quite primitive. We have today many tools and sources that allow us to have a clearer concept, although we, too, have limits, as we are speaking of things we cannot grab with our hands.

What is important to us is to determine what part of our human system is able to produce extraordinary physical outcomes. Now the answer to the question we asked ourselves when we began to study Qigong—what controls the energy in the process?—seems to have a clear answer. It has to be a control element distinct from the body (matter) and from energy (soul). Therefore it is the spirit that should control those actions. And since the characteristics of the defined spirit coincide with many of those of the mind (as defined today), sometimes we could accept to use those terms interchangeably. I cannot please at the same time agnostics and religious people.

How can one explain that the soul, being energy and life sustaining force, cannot act or think like the human brain? Further, how can one explain that the spirit cannot perceive painful or pleasurable feelings, that its communication is nonverbal, and that it is controlling our body and energy? What could be made in order to prevent people from transposing their human experiences to planes where there is no time, no matter, and no space, nor the feelings of hatred, pain, revenge, and so on?

Generally speaking, agnostic scientists who reluctantly accept the existence of a nonmaterial human component, and to whom the word *spirit* suggests a religious connotation, use different names like "the mind" or "higher consciousness," both of which have been assigned the same characteristics of nonlocality and no temporality as previously defined for the spirit. Curiously, in the German language the words for "mind" and "spirit" are the same (*Geist*). The same occurs in French. Hence the new trend called philosophy of mind, which involves taking care of the so-called mind-body problem (which could be compared to the spiritual-body relationship in most religions).

Here we stand between two stools. First, the pure scientists refuse to use terms like *spirit* so as to not give a religious connotation to their works, and therefore they incorporate into their lexicon a lot of words that mean the same thing and refer to something that has the same characteristics. On the other hand, the religious of all faiths believe that talking about "the spirit" as a component of our human system and giving it the characteristics of a control element is an act of demystification, dropping its characteristic of sacred and mysterious. This goes against the basic tenet of many religions, which is the unquestioned acceptance of dogmas and archetypes, even though these go against the most elementary logic or against the scientific discoveries of the past two centuries. Incredibly many religious leaders are pleased when scientists avoid using the word *spirit*. In both fields the scientific and religious they are very protective of their own lexicon. It is quite impossible to find a compromising or balancing point between the scientific and religious concepts of spirit, mind, and consciousness. Religious philosophers base their sustained arguments on ancient texts undoubtedly written when scientific knowledge was quite primitive while scientists refuse to incorporate nonmaterial, ancient concepts into their explanations.

The concept of mind is understood in many different ways by many different cultural and religious traditions. Some see mind as a property exclusive to humans. The attributes that make up the mind are much debated; some people confuse it with memory and reasoning. And there is a blurred threshold region that includes mind and consciousness mixed with spirit characteristics.

Mind is defined as the human consciousness that originates in the brain and is manifested especially in thought, perception, emotion, will, memory, and imagination. (Here using *consciousness* to define mind is quite redundant). It is also defined as the collective conscious and unconscious processes in a sentient organism that direct and influence mental and physical behavior. Still another definition is that mind is the element of a person that enables him or her to be aware of the world and his or her experiences, to think and to feel—the faculty of consciousness and thought. But people coincide that mind or consciousness is not physically located anywhere in our body.

For some scientists it is clear that there is a difference between the disembodied concept of the mind and that of the brain, which is simply an instrument in the form of a physical organ of the human body. According to neuropsychology, all brain function halts permanently upon brain death. The mind fails to survive brain death and ceases to exist. In this context brain is a sub product of mental (brain) activity.

Understanding the relationship between the brain and the mind (mind-body problem) is one of the central issues in the history of philosophy. It is a challenging problem both philosophically and scientifically. Recently the brain was defined as a transducer, which is a device that transforms some types of energy into other types. It also processes sensory perceptions and transforms them into complex ideas and feelings with their related reactions.

In our daily life, we see examples of transducers such as microphones and speakers that transform air vibration energy into electrical signals or vice versa, a thermometer that transforms heat into mechanical energy by expanding the column of mercury, or electronic thermometers that convert heat energy into electrical signals. The cells of our body are also transducers that convert temperature, images, smells, sounds, tastes, and the like into electrochemical signals that are sent using neurotransmitters to the brain and processed there as feelings.

The spirit (*mind* for many, *consciousness* or *higher consciousness* for others) requires the brain to exist as a transducer because it is the only one that is able to transform the instructions and commands generated outside the material body into physical actions. During certain special states of brain activity, one can bypass the intermediary action of the brain as transducer and establish a direct contact with the control element (spirit) through completely different channels of communication and interaction. All procedures to act on matter at a distance are possible during an altered state of consciousness, which basically consists of disconnecting the brain and its data banks to act at a nonverbal level.

The mind concept, when not fully understood as equivalent to spirit but as a brain activity sub product, cannot exercise any control over energy, though frequently people erroneously use expressions like "mind control" or "control of mind over matter." Others are reluctant to use the term *mind*, considering it associated with reasoning; such individuals instead use the term *psi*. In principle *mind* is a synonym of *psyche*. But when people assign those characteristics of the spirit to the mind or psyche, they are talking about the same thing—the control exerted by a no corporeal entity over matter. The proof that it is not the reasoning mind that can exercise control over matter is that during normal activity or mental thinking, one cannot achieve any of the extraordinary effects attributed to Qigong and raja-yoga. Only during meditative or similar processes designed to avoid thinking or discursive action can one access an altered state of consciousness, where the control element (spirit) assumes characteristics considered by many to be abnormal or paranormal because they do not follow the patterns of the ordinary thinking process of the brain. The practice of qigong is inconceivable without a good control altering and bypassing the ordinary mental processes.

CHAPTER 12

Preemptive Applications: Health and Longevity

There is an old Chinese proverb that says, "The activity of any doctor is to cure diseases, but only the good doctor avoids or prevents them." In other words, "Better safe than sorry." This makes perfect sense because having a disease, regardless of how quickly it is cured, means experiencing pain, disability, and psychological distress. Humans have great fear of two things—illness and death. The first involves decreased capabilities and pain, and the second is the cessation of life and the possible pleasures associated with it, which is the complete and irreversible loss of affections and possessions.

In ancient times the average human life-span was very short; reaching forty was a real accomplishment, considering that people had to survive among so many predatory animals, human enemies, and the elements of nature. Life was a constant fight, so to wake up each day still alive was a triumph. What nowadays for us may be just a slight illness or injury in those days could have been the cause of death. I had an aunt who said that we all suffer from a disease that is incurable and deadly. She was referring to aging.

In countries with ancient cultures such as China and India, some people were reported to have lived far beyond the bounds of the average lifetime, which enabled them to be in touch with the two following generations and be able to tell stories to grandchildren, some of whom had already lost their parents. In China, these people were called *immortals* because they survived whole generations that had already gone, and people did not know how much longer they could last. These *immortals* could have reached ninety years or maybe a little more, which was an extraordinarily long time, far beyond the average life expectancy of those around them. For the people of that epoch, why these elders had not died like the others was inexplicable, and many thought they had escaped death permanently.

According to Hebrew Scriptures (Tanakh) and the Christian Old Testament, a character called Methuselah lived between 900 and 1000 years. His actual life-span is debatable: scholars believe the number was misinterpreted or mistranslated because months (complete lunar cycles) were turned into years. Thus means his age would have been around 96.9 years, which was still extremely long for that epoch. In China legends were generated about people who had lived hundreds or thousands of years, such as Cheng Tze Kuang in the mountains of Omei or Hsu Che in the Cheng Ching mountains, but there is no evidence that any person had been ever in contact with them.

When people realized that those elders were not really immortals but indeed died, although later than others, and also that they remained in good physical condition, they became curious to find out what had preserved them so long and so well. They asked about their eating habits and, in general, about almost everything these people did or didn't do and tried to copy or imitate them. When these elders, so far considered immortals, lived in religious communities where control over their activities was easier, their customs were imitated to such an extent that they often turned into rules of life so that others might achieve the same results.

By the method of trial and error, the ancient Chinese discarded certain possibly harmful foods and certain habits as well that could harm the body. People also created breathing and strengthening exercises that in some cases imitated the movements of animals, especially those considered strongest.

Nowadays, analyzing the possible causes of that longevity, we observe that while all of these individuals were more in touch with nature, ate healthier meals, and breathed cleaner air, not everyone lived for the same span of time. Undoubtedly one of the differences had to be genetic. But most important was the nonexistence of what we know today as stress or psychological stress. They knew neither the term nor the phenomenon, but their meditative practices automatically freed them of any possible stress. We can thus assume an association between meditative practices and physical strengthening exercises with a lower number of diseases and ailments and longer life in better condition. All these teachings became an essential part of Qigong in China and likewise in India for the people practicing raja-yoga and following the *Yoga Sutras*.

A critical and objective approach compels us to reject the ancient belief about the existence of immortal beings, but we recognize that there must have been a group of people who by certain practices such as Qigong, lived longer and healthier. In Taoist lamaseries is where this aspect was most praised and cultivated, and therefore longevity has been always associated with the Tao. A reputed old text, the *Tao Te Ching*,[72] whose author was Laozi (a name that translated means "old master"), summarized the wisdom of ancient people regarding longevity. Such longevity does not refer just to longer life, but to slowing down the speed of chronological aging and getting to the last years of life in such a condition that one will not be a hindrance or burden to others. It means living longer in good health, experiencing fewer aches, pains, and sufferings, which allows one to enjoy the small pleasures of life and the company of beloved ones.

Modern medicine has come to the same conclusions that Qigong did several centuries ago, and both agree that the formula for better health and longer life consists of three factors: the first is healthy eating, the second is moderate physical exercise, and the third is reduction of tension or stress. Now it is common to see advertisements for products

---

72 The *Tao Te Ching*, *Daodejing*, or *Dao De Jing*, can be translated as "The Classic/Canon of the Way/Path and the Power/Virtue."

and programs offering stress relief or stress management. The number of centenarians currently living in the world is amazing, and this profusion is mainly due to the awareness and application of the above factors. Many years ago I had the opportunity to attend a seminar with Dr. Deepak Chopra in Puerto Rico, and one of the topics discussed was longevity. He made reference to a group of scientists who visited a mountain village in the Caucasus, where elders had an average age of 110 years. The scientists were searching for the fountain of youth, as did Ponce de Leon in Florida. After arduous research they did not find any food that could be considered the cause of longevity, but they realized several things. The first was that even after a hundred years, the elders were still performing difficult tasks like carrying water jugs up mountain slopes. (Continuing to exercise at advanced ages, which in our Western culture, is inconceivable.) The second factor was that in fact their diet was balanced, with little or no intake of sugars (which were hard to get in the mountains) and reduced animal protein intake. But the third factor appeared to be the most important: they had a minimum level of stress due to the harmony that reigned in the village and the absence of predators or human enemies. To conclude his speech, Dr. Chopra said that we appeared to have been placed under a curse: we would be forced to work until the end of our days; otherwise we would get sick and die prematurely. I remember the way he summarized his teaching in one sentence: "To retire only to rest is sitting to die."

I worked for a Dutch company for several years. The main concern of employees there was to retire with benefits that would provide them a comfortable and happy retirement. But the manager of the factory, of Danish origin, told me of a disturbing trend: people were living an average of only just a few years after their retirement. It made no sense to have worked for so many years only to enjoy just a few.

When corporate executives further studied the problem, they realized that the first year of retirement was the best: people enjoyed good health and enjoyed being free from work commitments—for them it was like an extended vacation. The problems began in the second year when that vacation became too long and people generally became inactive at home, just reading or watching television. Retirees also presented a so-called holiday syndrome that resulted from not returning to work after the break. Retired people realized that they were already considered useless for being old and were like waste from the production process. In our Western culture, aging can induce shameful feelings associated with the loss of power, energy, and sexual appeal, and thoughts of the imminent arrival of death. But more traditional cultures respect the accomplishment of longevity. There elders are seen as worthy members of their society, possessors of invaluable life experience and wisdom.

In general, retired people besides their low physical activity, experience mental stress caused by the feeling of social rejection for being old and unfit to work. What's worse was that many of these people had been able to continue working some ten years more under the same conditions of physical and mental efficiency. In fact, European countries increased the retiring age (though they didn't do it for the welfare of retirees but for economic reasons and lack of relief generations).

The studies conducted by the Dutch company determined that the key to solving the problem of the premature death of the pensioners would be to stop their feelings of uselessness. So they reduced working hours in the period before retirement, after which these retirement-age individuals were assigned some kind of minor activity that, though of no productive importance to the company, would make them feel useful even after retiring. Such activities could be as simple as counting screws in a warehouse (with the excuse that it was important in order that production lines would not stop) or participating as spectators (called "consultants") in some meetings. These simple changes were able to increase the average life expectancy of retirees.

This experience has been repeated in many companies and organizations and has introduced the activity known as occupational therapy, which is meant to improve workers' physical and mental health through assigning work that may not be significantly profitable or necessary to the company. People not only remain physically active, but their minds stay alert and free of stress.

Certainly you cannot rule out a genetic component that influences longevity, as there are families in which for some reason all members die young while in other families members die older. But exceptions in both groups can be produced by different modes of life. For instance, a person genetically programmed to die at a relatively young age may extend life or live better by following the procedures outlined by Qigong and modern science, while one programmed to live longer can shorten his life or continue to exist with more suffering if he or she fails to follow the right living procedures.

Many people practice gymnastics, aerobics, yoga, or countless variations of martial arts. Many others practice exercises with names that have just recently joined our lexicon. In the United States, numerous physical exercises are promoted as marketable products. These generally go out of fashion very quickly and are soon replaced by something similar with a different name. The constant variety of machines and devices to develop certain muscles seems endless. On many occasions advertisers hire famous film or television performers using them as a façade to sell what amounts to more of the same thing. For many in this culture, the quest to improve the appearance of the physical body has been diverted to a morbid and excessive love of self, known as narcissism.

At the peak of this trend is bodybuilding, the development of the muscles to their maximum shape for no practical purpose or activity but just for the appearance and image. Many people engage in this activity with extreme fanaticism, sometimes devoting many hours a day to train, perhaps with the intention to win a bodybuilding contest and gain the admiration of their peers and competitors. This activity has a parallel marketing promotion that involves the sale of many chemical and food products, many of which end up causing irreversible collateral damage, as in the case of certain injected drugs and anabolic substances.

A counterpart to that group of people is another: people who neglect their bodies by subjecting them to extreme hardship and practically destroying them by treating them like disposable gowns. In countries like India, unfortunately, this group reaches great proportions because these individuals think this way of life will conduct them to enlightenment.

Fortunately, there is always a compromise. In this case, an intermediate group honors the old belief that anything in excess is harmful, even something as simple and harmless as drinking water. This moderate group of people make use of meditation and relaxation techniques to cultivate their minds. While they don't pay too much attention to their bodies, they don't neglect them, either. The technique of Qigong combines these two main streams, cultivating the mind and maintaining the body for better health and longevity. Balance is critical in this technique, but since the two elements are inseparable, taking care of the body and cultivate the mind go hand in hand.

Among the preventive applications of Qigong is qi massage, which is both curative and prophylactic (or preventive). Using qi massage for either purpose requires knowledge of anatomy, bones, muscles, nerves, and meridians (*jing*) as well as the acupuncture points (*xue*).

Qi massage should not be confused with the normal massage intended to relax the individual. It is, rather, an energy-enhancing massage. Nor should it be confused with what some call the laying on of hands, a maneuver that has been largely discredited due to the mistakes of some undertrained teachers of Japanese Reiki.

Neophytes, people who have no idea of what Qigong procedures are, could get a wrong idea based on mere observation of qi massage and the maneuvers made by Qigong healers. In the center of hands there is indeed a point called *laogong* by which advanced masters can emit external qi (wei chi) and apply it on certain acupuncture points. This produces an action similar to that of acupuncture needles and in some cases exceeds their properties. It likely originated when doctors who had formerly practiced acupuncture had troubles sticking needles in young children who were nervous and crying (although actually proper use of acupuncture needles does not produce any pain). To overcome this difficulty, they chose another procedure, one that we in the West call acupressure. Thus involves applying pressure on certain acupuncture points and is often accompanied by the emission of external qi.

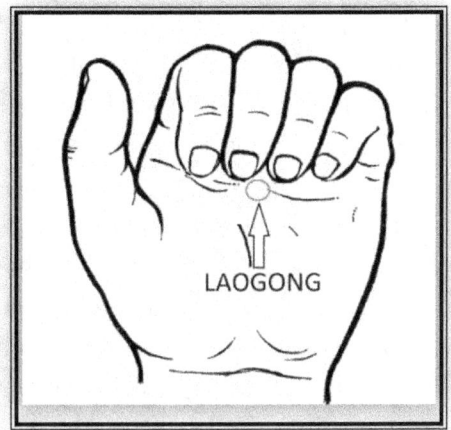

This type of massage, with some variations, served the martial arts performers who often suffered combat injuries in their practices. Performed by specialists, these massages combined the energy and analgesic functions with what today is called alignment—what chiropractors do to try to return muscles and bones to their original positions.

In case of severe trauma, Qigong can be of help, but it cannot repair a fracture or close an open wound immediately. I have personally attended injuries that could be handled with a qi-style massage combined with acupressure applied on pain-relief acupuncture sites. One morning as I was driving to my office, I witnessed a serious accident a hundred yards ahead of me. The driver appeared to have lost control. He'd hit the protection bars on the highway, and the car had bounced into the air, turning and landing upside down. I stopped ahead of the accident and got out of my vehicle, intending to call an emergency service from my cell phone.

When I approached the vehicle, I observed a middle-aged woman lying on the pavement. She looked unconscious or dead. People around did not dare to approach her; they watched from a distance. As I walked closer, I noticed that she was not bleeding. I touched her legs and arms to see if she had any fractures, and apparently there was none. She was still breathing, and her heart was beating. I told the other people who came near to not move the victim because she could have traumatized an organ or bone, and moving her without proper skill could cause a greater evil.

I did an emergency Qigong massage and she came to, but I ordered her not to move. The woman became conscious enough to speak clearly, with an Italian accent. She managed to give me the phone number of her daughter, whom I called. I told her what had happened, explaining also that firefighters would likely move her mother to a clinic or hospital, but I did not know where. The woman looked at me with eyes of surprise and said she felt no pain. She wanted to get up, to which I objected. I left her talking to paramedics from the fire department. They were surprised that a woman who had been ejected from a vehicle and beaten against the pavement was in such a condition of peace and consciousness. The use of Qigong in this case was highly effective, but only for the relief of posttraumatic pain; had the woman sustained a fracture, it would have been of little use, though perhaps it could have acted as an anesthetic to decrease the strong pain.

We do not know where massage came from as a human behavior, but it is an instinctive reaction to take hands to an area that hurts or has been traumatized, and we all have felt the difference. Possibly our body knows at an unconscious level that the action of the hands relieves pain.

Qigong massage and self-massage (an-mo) have four types. The first, *pu tong an mo*, is a general massage that produces relaxation and stimulates peripheral circulation. It does not differ much from traditional Western massage, except that it often includes a transfer of external qi and the application of pressure to acupuncture areas. Some argue that this type of massage also helps to strengthen the immune system and extend longevity. These effects have been confirmed in laboratories, since the pressure on certain points stimulates secretion of endorphins that relieve pain and increase the immune response. The second type is tui *na an mo* (massage pressure and grip), and the third is *dian xue an mo* (massage pressure on acupuncture cavities), similar to Japanese Shiatsu. These two last types of therapeutic massage are to be applied by a doctor or specialist, as their misuse or misapplication may produce harmful side effects. And finally the fourth type is *qi an mo* (qi energy massage), which for many is considered more of a medical treatment than a massage.

Although Qigong massage provides relief and healing, sometimes its therapeutic action is not as fast as that of (invasive) Western medical treatments. However, it offers some advantages in that it corrects problems at their source and in a natural way. These massages do not produce side effects, nor do they require the use or ingestion of chemicals that could be harmful in the long run.

These massages can also be combined with other techniques, such as ingestion or application of herbs, pressure with hot and cold stones, acupuncture, and moxibustion[73]. Though not a very common technique, application of lotions or oils is sometimes used. Often to prevent skin irritation from the friction or pressure, a soft towel of silk or cotton is placed between the hands of the practitioner and the patient. In some cases small devices are incorporated, such as porcelain, timber, or padded rollers; balls of metal or stones; thin metal rods shaped like brushes (for tapping); and even small hammers. Most of these gadgets or tools are not used in the previously mentioned types of massages but are included in *muscle/tendon changing* or the Qigong *bone-marrow cleansing*, two methods for increasing the superior physical resistance to impacts received especially in the martial arts.

---

73 This is a traditional Chinese medicine therapy using moxa made from dried mugwort. There are several methods of moxibustion. Three of them are direct scarring, direct nonscarring, and indirect moxibustion. Direct scarring moxibustion places a small cone of mugwort on the skin at an acupuncture point and burns it until the skin blisters, which then scars after it heals. Direct nonscarring moxibustion removes the burning mugwort before the skin burns enough to scar, unless the burning mugwort is left on the skin too long. Indirect moxibustion, probably the most common, holds a cigar made of mugwort near the acupuncture point to heat the skin or holds it on an acupuncture needle inserted in the skin to heat the needle.

CHAPTER 13

Qigong and Sexuality

The Chinese friend of mine who worked at the embassy sent his wife to China for three months so she would be available to help her daughter prepare for admission exams to enter a well-reputed primary school. In China, as in Japan, to enter the best schools and universities is very hard; thus those entering a good primary school almost have a guarantee to access to a reputable high school and then a well-known university. For this reason preparation to be admitted into the primary educational institutions is very important. I asked my friend if such a lengthy separation from his family caused him discomfort, to which he replied that, on the contrary, it was very good. He explained that his qi would be increased during this period because he would conserve the energy typically lost during their intimate relationships.

We cannot deny that a waste of energy occurs during a sexual intercourse, but it also occurs when we run or do some strenuous exercise. Of course, during sexual activity there is an additional energy transfer with the contribution of the male sperm, which is composed of living cells endowed with much energy and surrounded by a transporting medium rich in proteins and vitamins[74]. The Chinese claim that during

---

74   In addition to spermatozoids (2% to 5%), the male semen contains fructose (2–5 mg per mL, the main energy source of sperm cells), amino acids, citrate, enzymes, flavins, phosphorylcholine, prostaglandins, proteins, vitamin C, acid phosphatase, citric acid, fibrinolysin, prostate-specific antigen, proteolytic enzymes, and zinc (whose level is about 135±40 micrograms/ml for healthy men).

sexual intercourse, there is a transfer of an essence (*jing* 精) that one should attempt not to waste but to develop and accumulate. That *jing*, being a sexual energy, is considered to dissipate with ejaculation, so masturbation is considered energy suicide among those who practice qiqgong. However, with adequate rest and good nutrition, the human body is able to restore its energy balance. It is important to note that we are talking about a moderate rate of sexual activity, since any excessive activity wears the body down by not giving it time enough to recover; furthermore, that excess can be harmful when combined with poor nutrition, lack of rest, drinking, and smoking.

Since much of the knowledge on Qigong comes from convents and monasteries, where teachings were transferred from experienced monks to novices and where sexual activity was generally prohibited, many people have associated sexual restriction with practicing Qigong. However Confucius (Kong Zi) clarified that "Both hunger and sexuality are natural feelings of man and a total ban on sexuality, especially for a long time, could be maintained only by very few people with a great deal of perseverance."

Common to all living beings are birth, growth, reproduction, and death. To perpetuate the animal species, these make use of multiple methods, the most common being the fertilization of a cell (ovum) in the recipient female by a cell (sperm) from the fertilizing male. In lower animals such as flatworms and amoebas, one can observe asexual reproduction by division; these creatures reach their normal size after having been divided into two halves. In order that fertilization and sexual reproduction can be achieved, however, there must be an attraction (as pleasure) between male and female. The odds that sexual intercourse could occur randomly are remote, and it is only thanks to the attraction between opposite sexes and the pleasure that sexual intercourse gives to both sides that the majority of animal species can be perpetuated.

The thinking and rational human capacity, combined with more free time and leisure in modern society, has caused us to circumvent the cycles of nature (mating season in females) and look for satisfaction or sexual pleasure detached from procreation, its primary purpose. That pursuit of pleasure, just for the pleasure itself, has given rise to acts of lust and deviations of all kinds. We understand lust as the sublimation of sexual pleasure in itself and the search to achieve that satisfaction by any means. So today we see that the pornography industry has become a multimillion-dollar business, and nearly all promotion of normal (nonsexual) products includes a subliminal sexual message.

It is appropriate to clarify certain aspects of Qigong as they relate to sexuality. Among people who practice Qigong, one can undoubtedly find a stream of celibate individuals who say that sexual acts are a waste of vital energy that can deplete or harm the body, and thus these individuals promote sexual restriction and prefer to follow a kind of monastic life. Perhaps this behavior is related to the history of Chinese emperors and feudal lords, who usually had many concubines. That conduct was mainly enacted for reasons of status and social level; that is, it was only a visible accumulation of females to show off their possessions (the way some Arabian kings did). It is historically documented that among an emperor's many concubines, there were some he never touched. Sometimes when the emperor visited a province, he brought as a concubine one of the governor's daughters to flatter the governor and make him feel part of the royal court, but he did not mean to have sexual intercourse with the maid. The emperor had some concubines with whom he did have carnal relations, but he had limit such in order to avoid exhaustion, especially when entering his mature years. Most of the medical advisers to the ruling emperor suggested that he reduce his frequency of sexual intercourse. In many cases they advised the emperor to have sex but avoid ejaculation so as to not waste his vital energy. They said that a drop of semen was equal to ten drops of blood, so it should not be wasted. They even advised him to press with his fingers on certain acupuncture points to stop or retard ejaculation.

These concepts of conservation of vital energy have been transferred to the present day, and some follow them with a fanatic attitude. However, the best approach is to achieve a balance between excess and total restriction. Moderate sex is neither draining nor harmful.

Qigong masters advise apprentices not to drill for a brief period after having sex. These tips are based on experience: masters would observe pupils who lacked energy only to find out that they had just had sex. But one does not need to be a scholar to realize this phenomenon. A period of rest is advisable to allow the body to automatically restore its previous levels. In cases of people who practice Qigong to produce healing, the situation is more delicate because they can hardly accumulate energy and then transmit it if their own levels are depleted or inadequate.

It is important to not treat the lessons of ancient Qigong as dogma because over time these teachings have undergone modifications and adaptations as a result of experience, which parallels the development of other sciences. I've seen pictures of ancient Qigong followers in which they hanged heavy weights to the testes and the member. These activities might be typical of ignorant people in ancient times, but today they have no place and should be avoided at all costs. We must always bear in mind that the human is an evolving animal that should make use of others' accumulated past experiences so as to avoid repeating their mistakes.

The ancient Chinese described a process of transformation of the *jing essence* (human sperm) into qi energy. For them it seemed logical that human sperm, like urine and feces, were products that should come out of the body and not build up inside. Many texts located the sperm generation in the kidneys, since according to their observations, it was in that organ that urine was formed, a substance that goes out through the same hole in males. They noticed as well that during periods of abstinence, it seemed that sperm accumulated, and irrespective of time this accumulation disappeared internally, especially when they practiced certain Qigong exercises. Therefore they attributed disappearance to the transformation of the jing into qi. They obviously were very far from knowing the physiological processes that allow the reabsorption or elimination of sperm by automatic means[75]. But they really were not that wrong because when energy (in the form of fructose and other substances) does not go outside and get reabsorbed, some type of energy conservation does in fact take place.

Nature in its wise mechanisms for preservation of the species makes just the fittest and strongest the ones to reproduce. Thus we observe the behavior of the so-called dominant males or alpha males in groups of lower animals, which does not allow that weaker or sick animals be able to reproduce. Nature also has provisions for animals not to reproduce when environmental conditions are unfavorable, such as natural disasters, imminent danger from predators, and especially before food shortages, situations that in human modern societies have been replaced by stress derived from situations of economic or social difficulties. As the practice of Qigong is a method to replenish and increase energy levels, within certain limits, it is logical that the body in favorable conditions may be more prone to seek reproduction and sexual mating.

It has been scientifically proven that the practice of Qigong stimulates the secretion of hormones in the adrenals and the release of endorphins and catecholamine, which creates a feeling of wellness that affects the sexual appetite. Because of this the masters prevent their disciples from wasting energy by citing the example of a person who wishes to fill a bucket of water that has some holes in the bottom—regardless of the amount of water poured into the bucket, one will not succeed in filling it completely.

When we are charged with vital energy by practicing Qigong, we must not allow deterioration caused by excessive sexual practices; we must seek a balance, especially if we have not reached the optimal energy level. This optimal level could be defined by taking into account certain characteristics, such as moderate reduction of appetite (i.e., feeling satisfied by what you eat even if it is not very abundant) and a feeling that the body is lighter, almost as if it is floating in the air. In addition,

---

75 Phagocytosis of old spermatozoids by Sertoli cells.

the mind will feel clear and perceptive, and senses will be enhanced: vision will cover the whole field of view (to 180 degrees), smells will be more subtle and tastes more varied, sounds will be perceived from great distances and more clearly, and paranormal abilities (telepathy, clairvoyance, and the like) will be enhanced as well.

CHAPTER 14

Healing Procedures with Subtle Energy

The history of humankind is full of reports of unexplainable healings, some of them labeled as miracles. At this time in the twenty-first century, advances in the medical sciences, biology, and related areas are paramount; nevertheless people still continue to report healings that occur without the use of conventional medicine.

For scientists this is a debatable topic full of contradictions. Many explanations have been provided for this extended phenomena. I am not a scientist or researcher and cannot give answers to many questions. But for a specialized opinion, I will refer to that of Dr. Gary E. Schwartz, PhD, who wrote the following:

> *"I'm a Harvard PhD, a former Yale professor of psychology and psychiatry and director of the Yale Psychophysiology Center. I'm currently a professor of psychology, surgery, medicine, neurology and psychiatry at the University of Arizona. I was awarded one of two NIH grants to establish a Center for Frontier Medicine in Biofield[76] Science. Though I was originally taught that such healing miracles do not and cannot happen, the fact is that they do. Science can now help us to understand and celebrate them."*

Extensive scientific analysis on this topic is beyond the scope of this book, but for the reader who is interested in going deeper into this theme, I recommend a classic book on this subject: *The Energy Healing Experiments: Science Reveals Our Natural Power to Heal.*[77]

But it is worth differentiating having the *capacity* to heal and being *able* to heal. In principle all humans have the capacities to perform many things in the areas of athletics, science, the arts, and more. The problem lies in how to develop these capacities. And the worst thing is when someone presumes to have extraordinary healing capacities (who really does not) and takes advantage of others for personal gain.

Another related problem are the people who by ignorance or unjustified pride assume functions of voluntary healers but produce no results or, in some cases, producing further progression of an illness. We have seen people who, overconfident after participating in a short weekend seminar on the laying on of hands (again, different and detached from Qigong), tried to conduct healing, believing they had acquired supernatural healing powers that in fact existed only in their fantasy. There have been many reported cases about mistakes made by

---

76 Biofield therapies are intended to affect energy fields that purportedly surround and penetrate the human body. The existence of such fields has not yet been scientifically proven. Some forms of energy therapy manipulate Biofields by applying pressure and/or manipulating the body by placing the hands in, or through, these fields.

77 See *The Energy Healing Experiments* by Gary E. Schwartz, PhD, with William L. Simon (New York: Atria Books, 2007) ISBN-13:978-0-7432-9237-5.

such pseudo-healers. Unfortunately, they do not have a malpractice insurance policy. I knew firsthand of a friend's twelve-year-old daughter who had a strong pain in the lower abdomen, a symptom of a medical problem. The family, instead of taking her to a hospital, tried to heal her with only their good intentions and their hands. Due to the thus time wasted, what had been the beginning of appendicitis turned into a severe case of peritonitis. Our grandparents had a beautiful saying in Spanish that translated goes, "Do not try to be a witch doctor if you don't have a previous knowledge on herbs." People should be warned in order not to fall in the hands of charlatans or quacks.

For many years scientists around the world held the belief that the human immune system could not be controlled externally, that it was autonomous. However, a scientist, Dr. David L. Felten[78] discovered that human nerve fibers were in fact connected to both the immune system and the nervous system. From that idea and others associated with it, a new branch of medical science called psycho-neuro-immunology has emerged. Research in this area serves to explain why systems like Qigong are able to affect hormone levels, healing, and pain control in humans.

Dr. Higucchi,[79] in his article "Endocrine Immune Response during 'Qi-Gong' Meditation," reported on experiments conducted on two groups of people, one group practicing Qigong, and the other a control group. After meditating for an hour, most of the Qigong group showed increases in endorphin levels. But surely the best proof is what we experience in ourselves that allows us to feel firsthand a substantial improvement of our health and well-being.

The historical narrative of the Christian Bible that appears in the New Testament is based on the so-called public life of Jesus of Nazareth. It is basically a recount of his teachings, or parables, and his miracles and wonders. The Catholic religion encourages the so-called cult of the

---

78 David L. Felten, MD, is a well-known and respected researcher whose contributions helped to establish the field of psycho-neuro-immunology and lay the foundations for the physiological understanding of complementary and integrative medicine.

79 See "Endocrine and Immune Response During Qi-gong Meditation," *Journal of International Society of Life Information Science* (vol.14, no.2, 1996).

miracles, giving more importance to miracles than to many other things, and so appoints, or canonizes, each year new saints, mainly based on their miracles. The religion also encourages and promotes pilgrimages to holy places such as Fatima in Portugal and Lourdes in France, where the primary objective of the participants is to obtain miraculous cures (while the tours organizers gain economic benefit).

In this religion the primary function of a saint is that of mediation before God in order that the faithful be granted miracles. In principle this religion never accepts that it is the saint who performed the miracle: he or she is just an instruments of God. After death these saints supposedly become agents or brokers who intercede before God for the petitioner to achieve a miracle. If it cannot be proved without a doubt that the intervention of some pious deceased person produced a miracle, he or she will only be remembered as a good person—and soon forgotten. But if according to the petitioner, the intervention achieved a miraculous cure, then the saint-to-be will begin to climb the ladder to his or her holiness, first passing through the degree of blessed or venerable. So sanctification is paradoxically dependent on the petitioners, who always do their requests or petitions to the saint or dead person who has a reputation for being more effective. No one asks miracles of my deceased grandfather, so he never will be a holy saint, but to Pope John Paul II, being a figure known to all, there will be many who will solicit miracles and place him on the ladder to sure sanctification[80].

In this way a culture and generation of miracle seekers has been created (we even expect miracles from politicians). We are all beggars at different levels. All the temples are filled with petitioners to a greater or lesser extent. Once the so-called saints are "ascended to the altar"

---

80 The original of this book published in Spanish some years ago presented this as a hypothesis for something that could happen in the future, but John Paul II's cause for canonization commenced in 2005 shortly after his death with the traditional five year waiting period waivered. On 19 December 2009, John Paul II was proclaimed Venerable by his successor Pope Benedict XVI and was beatified on 1 May 2011 after the Congregation for the Causes of Saints attributed one miracle to him, the healing of a French nun from Parkinson's disease. A second miracle, attributed to the late pope, was approved on 2 July 2013 and confirmed by Pope Francis two days later. John Paul II was canonised on 27 April 2014.

(i.e., become subject of veneration), then starts the process of prayers, candles, requests, and promises for miraculous solutions. Most of the petitioners, when they are not satisfied, go to another instance (another saint). People summarized this activity of the Catholic Church with a popular Spanish saying: "When there are new saints, the old ones cannot perform any more miracles!"

During my childhood I was educated in a Catholic school, but when I reached adulthood, I was surprised to be informed that "miracles" had occurred not only in my religion but also in many other religions and cults; in this way I became aware that we did not have the exclusive rights to such! It seemed unreal the first time I read about the Tibetan monks, sadhus of India, Buddhist monks, dervishes, Sufi Islam, Rabbis, and even aboriginal shamans and warlocks in Africa and America. All had made wonders equivalent to those of our Catholic saints, but they were not yet ascended to the heavens and were not revered, much less used as agents or brokers for further miracles.

Inexplicable cures, according to traditional medicine, have been reported in other cultures: though the healing methods were different, the events were similar. After studying them, we can see that they are based on the same energy-controlling principles. For example, in Japan there is a healing procedure that is known as Reiki, which is based on the very same concept of universal life energy. The Japanese word *ki* is the equivalent of the Chinese *qi*. So Reiki can be compared with the Qigong Liao Fa, which is the branch applied to healing physical ailments.

Followers of Reiki in Japan and overseas attribute the rediscovery of this energy in their country to a Christian monk named Usui Mikao, who was the principal (Abbot) of a Christian monastery in Tokyo in the late nineteenth century. (Remember that Qigong precedes this by several centuries). This monk was rebuked by his students, who demanded to know why they were not learning anything about the healing systems used by Jesus of Nazareth and why their teacher could not make such a demonstration of power, questions the monk was unable to respond to at that time. It is said that in his search to answer those challenging questions, he went to the United States, where he studied for a doctorate in theology at the University of Chicago. He complained that in the Christian scriptures, there were no teachings of the healing method of placing on of hands. Because of his ability to speak Japanese, Chinese, English, and Sanskrit, he continued his search until he rediscovered some Sanskrit formulas and symbols in Buddhist scriptures that seemed to give answer to his concern. From then onward he began teaching, preaching, and healing, and his main disciple was Dr. Chijiro Hayashi (who died in 1941).

Reiki (after long training and preparation) when applied properly tends to replicate the same effects of Qigong Liao Fa, as they work on the same principle of vital energy. The problem with the training of Reiki is that currently it is made very superficial and commercial, teaching just the body parts where one should place the hands for a particular ailment. Attempts to sell merchandise ignore the fact that to manipulate life energy, the healer (preferably a physician) must be thoroughly trained. Also ignored is that Reiki is to be applied only during an altered state of consciousness, and this also requires long and strict training. I attended two Reiki courses in Miami, Fla., where most of the participants were people linked to physiotherapy, massage, and the like. These courses sought in weekend seminars to teach a complicated and ancient procedure, and certainly the goal of the organizers was to make money. Participants were lying on of hands while amiable chatting which is not the real procedure.

One flaw in those who correctly practice Reiki is a kind of veneration of their masters, those who restarted this science in Japan. At the beginning of a healing session practitioners contact these masters, imploring for protection and assistance, not unlike what Catholics ask of their saints, turning that technique into a pseudo religion.

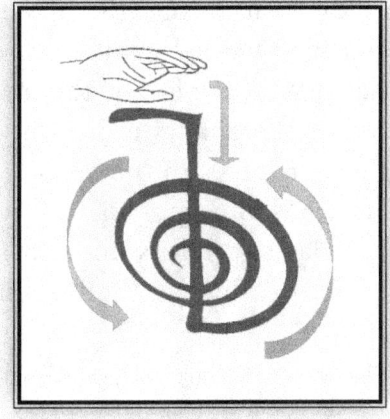

Another anomaly of this teaching is the use of certain graphic symbols (derived from Japanese characters) to which magical or miraculous properties are attributed when hands move along following those patterns.

This goes so far as to induce followers to use these symbols by drawing them in the air with their hands over food and gifts as well as using them in a letter to be sent far away to remotely cure a person. We should understand that it is undisputed that a cure can be effected remotely however, it cannot be done by using superficial, almost magical, methods.

Another school that applies this type of energy to conduct healing is the Pranic Indian School, which controls and uses prana, the Indian equivalent of qi. The technique is called pranic healing. It is said to be a therapy in human biological fields[81] (similar to magnetic fields of the planet) and also seems to have originated in China thousands of years ago, only to be "rediscovered" in more modern times by Mei Ling (sixth century AD) and Choa Kok Sui (twentieth century AD). Pranic Healing has been registered as a trademark by Choa Kok Sui[82], and it has been quite discredited by the commercial use of its procedures. But in principle it is considered a medical application of subtle energies in which followers claim to use prana, universal force, or life-force to promote or encourage healing. Pranic Healing, as described by its supporters, is based on observation conducted by certain sensitive subjects who are able to perceive the so-called energy fields, or auras of different colors, around the human body. A healer's ability to see auras falls within the clairvoyant abilities. These healers say that the color of the aura and the energy centers, or chakras, reflect the changing health status of the body. They describe three steps or stages in the healing process. In the first, the healer imparts blessings and appreciation to the masters who have given guidance (similar to what is done in Reiki healing). In the second stage, the healer conducts a kind of energy scan in the aura of the subject to

81 There is a new area of scientific studies known as biofields. Some researchers affirm that all alternative healing therapies act on those fields that are located around the physical body.

82 The Pranic Healing brand-name is a registered trademark of the Institute for Inner Studies Inc., a for-profit company founded by Choa Kok Sui.

diagnose any abnormalities. Finally the healer cleans and energizes the body, the chakras, and the aura (Biofield?) of the subject. But regardless of the rituals associated and the sequence of the process, the important thing is that these practitioners are working with the same energy the Chinese call qi. And although regarded by some as a pseudo medicine, Pranic Healing should instead be considered an alternative medicine.

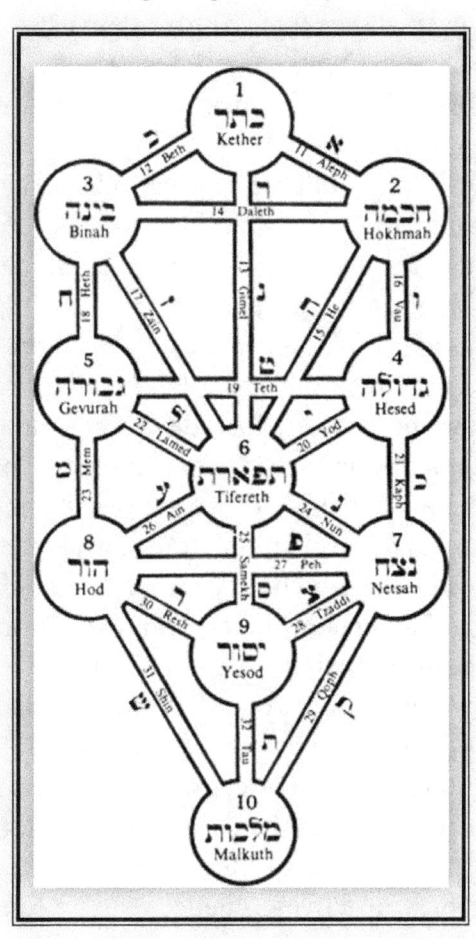

In another culture, Judaism, Kabbalah is a school that refers to mental influences and intentional promotion in the areas of the chain of being. Within this context Kabbalah healing is considered a spiritual healing (accomplished by means not attributable to a physical action) based on ancient Kabbalah knowledge. This procedure runs well whether the patient is present or distant. Practitioners define it as a mental influence within the context of their sacred Kabbalah, through which the healer is able to have an effect on the physical and mental condition of the patient[83].

People generally recognize that the principles and mechanisms of remote healing have not yet been adequately clarified by scientists.

83 Luria, I. (1988a). "Eytz Chaim" (The tree of life). In C., Vital (Ed.), *Kitvei Ari* (Writings of Ari) (Vol. 1–2). Jerusalem: Vedebsky. Luria, I. (1988b). "Shaar HaKavonos" (The gate of mental intentions). In C., Vital (Ed.), *Kitvei Ari* (Writings of Ari), Jerusalem: Vedebsky.

However, Bell's theorem[84] seems to prove their effectiveness, since in Qigong healing also operates remotely with equal results. According to Bell, the actions of the mind (or the spirit) in an altered state of consciousness are timeless and nonlocal (outside the space-time dimension). Ancient rabbis dominated mental influence for the purpose of spiritual growth, healing, and helping others. The most publicized remote healing was recorded in the Christian Bible when Jesus healed a centurion's slave in Capernaum, a city of Galilee at a distance, without physical approaching him. (Luke 7:1–10 and Matthew 8:5–13).

The Kabbalistic healers allege that (like Qigong), their procedure can improve any physical or mental condition, including chronic illnesses and those for which traditional medicine has been limited or ineffective. They also allege that it improves living conditions such as is accomplished as well by prophylactic or preventive Qigong.

During the Kabbalah healing process, two rabbis serve the patient simultaneously. In order to be able to exercise a mental influence, the practitioner needs to engage in an "intentional mental ascent" (*kavonah*) to higher levels of existence, which in modern scientific terms equals access to an altered state of consciousness. The rabbis define this condition as one in which perceptions are different from those in our normal life, and as a result the practitioner cannot engage in verbal communication with the patient while he is under mental influence because doing so would cause a return to normal consciousness and spoil the treatment. Qigong is performed in much the same way: while the master implements his treatment, he is in an altered state of consciousness and cannot talk to the patient or perform other activities. The rabbis in such state are able to identify negative influences known as *klipos* (covers). These negative influences can be conscious or unconscious and include

---

84[*] Bell's theorem states that the concept of local realism, favored by Einstein, yields predictions that disagree with those of quantum mechanical theory. Because numerous experiments agree with the predictions of quantum mechanical theory and show correlations that are, according to Bell, greater than could be explained by local hidden variables, the experimental results have been taken by many as refuting the concept of local realism as an explanation of the physical phenomena under test.

depression (*marah schorah*), impulsivity (*marah lavonah*), anxiety (*daygos*), egocentricity (*yeshus*), and arrogance (*gayvah*). Coincidentally, scientific research shows that cognitive and emotional processes can be conscious or unconscious[85].

In the Islam faith, there is a group of believers that, according to interpretation of the Holy Koran, do not accept spiritual (mind) healing or in general any intervention by Allah. However, another esoteric group of Islam, known as Sufis (Tasawwuf) accepts and uses healing procedures that control universal energy. Attributed to them are what in ancient times and even in the modern era are called healing miracles. Their procedures, too, are initiated by rituals that provide access to an altered state of consciousness. In the case of the dervishes, for example, this is achieved by turning the body in multiple rounds of dances.

The Spanish of the period in which Granada was liberated from Muslim rule had a very nice saying: "Do the miracle! Even if it is Muhammad who does it!" which meant that they cared about the result and not the instrument, because by that time they had realized that Christians were not the only ones who performed miracles. An account of miracles performed in non-Christian faith that caught my attention was that of a writer named Abdul-Hadi, who recorded more than six centuries ago what his father said to him one day:

"You were born as a result of a prayer of the great Bahaudin Naqshband of Bokhara, whose miracles are innumerable" Years after, Bahaudin explained to Abdul: "Now, about that which you call miracles all here have seen miracles. What is important is the function of miracles. Miracles can be designed to provide a portion of the food which is an extra meal, and can act on the mind and even on the body in a certain sense. When this happens, the experience of the miracle made its own proper function in the mind. If the miracle acts only on the imagination of the

---

85 Winkielman, P., Berridge, K. C., & Wilbarger, J. (2005). "Emotion, Behavior, and Conscious Experience: Once More without Feeling." In L.F. Barrett, P.M. Niedenthal, & P. Winkielman (eds.), *Emotion and Consciousness* (pp. 335–362). New York: Guilford Press.

mind as raw mentality it encourages uncritical credulity or emotional excitation, or a thirst for more miracles, or a desire to understand the miracles, or a biased affection toward the person who performed the miracle or even the fear of him.[86]"

> ## "The candle is not there to illuminate itself."
> ## Nawab Jan-Fishan Khan

Based on miracles, there are many who should be considered Christian saints, but they belong to Sufism. Among them are Cheik Halladj Mansour (921–922), the alchemist Djabir Ibn Hayyan, Ibrahim ibn Adham, Yahya al Razi, and Ibn Fudhayl Iyadh[87].

Sufi spiritual healers imagine or represent the flow of life-force in the body and in the universe as energy vortexes composed of a group of even smaller spirals, or cones of energy. These are known in Islamic terminology as *lat'if*, meaning "subtle manifestations" or "layers." The *lata'if* (singular *latiifa*) are the points of maximum energy intake and focal points of balance considered very important in the energetic system. Diseases and illnesses are thought to occur if a *latiifa* is unbalanced. Depending on the Sufi order or group, there are small differences in the location and color of the *lata'if*. The *zikr*, simply translated as "divine remembrance" is also practiced as a method to cure mental and physical illnesses. The procedure is conducted by repetition of sacred verses, individually or in groups, usually under the supervision of a Sufi master.

After having examined Eastern cultures and the other two Judeo-Christian religions (Judaism and Islam), we cannot disregard the healing procedures conducted by Christian confessions. We should mention the Christian Pentecostals and Catholics Charismatics who basically incorporate healing rituals within the broad spectrum of Christian faiths.

---

86 *The Sufis* by Idries Shah. New York: Anchor Press Books (Doubleday), 1964.
87 *La Puerta: Sufismo, Ediciones Obelisco*, Barcelona, España, 1988.

Original Pentecostal churches, also called classical, are made up of clusters of evangelical Christians whose purpose is to proclaim the Gospel of Jesus Christ to all nations by performing miracles, healings, and other demonstrations sponsored by the Holy Spirit. Pentecostalism has grown but divided, so it is possible to find numerous small churches and denominations apparently unconnected but following similar principles. There are more than twenty different major Pentecostal branches, and it is reported that altogether there are several million followers. In Catholicism, Pentecostalism is known as Charismatic Renewal, with a growing number of followers.

Both denominations include in their healing ceremonies the control of vital energy (qi), considered by them a divine energy from the Holy Spirit. Their ceremonies include the imposition (laying on) of hands. No doubt some healings must have been successful because their rituals include access to an altered state of consciousness, and if had it not been so, the followers would had dispersed. I had the opportunity to attend a Pentecostal ceremony in the city of Fort Valley, Georgia, where the minister was so admired that many who had Pentecostal's temples nearer to their homes made the long journey to that place. In the ceremony I could see a charged atmosphere of euphoria when certain hymns were sung, at the end of which at times the minister conducted the laying on of hands.

No doubt ministers should have succeeded in achieving healings or cures in those Pentecostal and Charismatic Christian temples, for they work on the confirmed energy-control principles. However, sometimes in these groups (but not always) parishioners have been manipulated for proselytizing purposes. A church in Brazil (that does not belong to either of the above-mentioned faiths) has been reported to be doing big business with its alleged cures. They profusely broadcast commercial-type promotions in TV. People attend the ceremonies looking for relief from their pains, and they leave the temple with empty pockets and purses. Many well-documented studies about their conduct have been published, and many complaints have reached the courts.

There are many skeptics of simple cures used for proselytizing purposes (in any religion or group), and they allege two types of discrediting explanations. The first is related to so-called spontaneous healings generated by the self-defense mechanisms of the human body. This argument states that the illness in question, such as influenza or an infectious disease, would have been cured anyway, regardless of what the priest or minister was able to do. This effect is also known as a circumstantial connotation or the *rain dance* effect. In the past in Native American tribes, when the dry season became unbearable and rains were very close but had not yet arrived, the Indians danced to their gods to bring rain. It was enough that one single time, coincidentally, it rained after they'd danced: this created the dance-rain association. Furthermore, over time, as usually these dances were performed at the end of the summer's dry season, the positive outcomes were likely repeated several times, to the point that the people began considering the dance as the sole cause of the rain. In short, it is a fact that people take credit for natural events over which they have had no supernatural influence or control. This behavior is also observed in healers and shamans who do not belong to an organized religion.

The second explanation that discredits those actions is the placebo effect, whereby any person may experience genuine pain relief through self-suggestion. When doctors introduce a new experimental drug, to be sure of their results, they administer the medicine to two different groups of people. One group (the control) receives the drug while the other receives a placebo—nothing more than a simulation of the drug. Of course, neither of the groups knows what is being given to them; they all think they are getting the real drug. The ones who get the placebo generally receive pills or tablets containing harmless substances (a glucose powder or lozenge or other nontherapeutic component), and when injections are required, they receive harmless aqueous dilutions. After the experiment, the results are compared, and they can be surprising. Some people who were given the placebo but were convinced of the potential effect of the new drug healed as if they'd received the real medicine dose. In well-documented cases physicians have reported that they administered injections of an aqueous solution to patients with severe pain while telling them that it was a powerful new painkiller, and the pain disappeared. Other physicians have applied creams that only contained a fat base to patients with skin disorders, and those problems disappeared as well. In other cases, patients with frequent colds were given what they were told were massive doses of vitamin C, when in fact they only got sugar water; still the frequency of their colds decreased substantially.

It is interesting to remark that this placebo effect, that continues to baffle doctor, has been reported only in human beings. It does not work on plants or irrational animals. In similar laboratory tests conducted on pairs or groups of plants or mice, the results differ substantially. Probably because none of these groups could be induced or is prone to suggestion.

Something like the placebo effect was used to defend a Pentecostal minister in a congregation where it was reported that cures were fraudulent or simulated. The minister claimed that these false cures were introduced and proclaimed in order to strengthen the faith of the participants and thus later on possibly bring about true healings.

The worst cases of fraud have been observed in the televangelists, who have television shows on which they make people believe they are performing cures in the name of God, or by expelling demons out of the bodies of the patients. These cures are really deceptions of various kinds. Their methods range from using radio transmission to provide the patient's data to the celebrant or searching for people with less severe illnesses, such as people who have to use a wheelchair but have not totally lost the ability to walk.

When the authorities of the US Internal Revenue Service audited these televangelists, they detected fabulous personal incomes that in many cases exceed $800,000 per year, excluding other perks. In another country, a messenger belonging to a religious organization from Brazil was assaulted while carrying hundreds of thousands of dollars in cash obtained from parishioners in search of alleged cures. Thereafter their bishops hired a security service (escorts or bodyguards) in order to not suffer any more theft, blackmailing, or kidnapping, though once one of them was detained at US customs for carrying a lot of cash that had not been declared and could not be justified. A book entitled *The Faith Healers*[88] documents many cases of this kind, which continue to occur. Unfortunately the victims are mostly people who already had serious health problems and whose funds that otherwise could be used for regular medical treatments are now depleted with no results.

In addition some ministers of different faiths start a so-called cascade effect by telling their parishioners about miraculous cures that only they (the ministers) had witnessed. Thereafter the members of the congregation repeat the story as if they had been present, and a lie repeated a thousand times becomes a truth. A self-critical Pentecostal said he had never seen anyone restore sight to the blind, heal a leper, raise the dead, make a paralytic walk, or perform any of the other miracles attributed to Jesus of Nazareth. What he *had* seen were cases of temporary relief of minor ailments.

Any group, sect, or religion that uses supposed miraculous cures for propaganda purposes is subject to continued dishonest practices in order to keep its customers flowing. The Christian narrative of Jesus's healings never once mentions that he charged anything or received compensation of any kind. Perhaps that's why many of these mercantile-oriented groups use terms like *donation, contribution,* and so forth to disguise the real plunder.

From the very moment that fees, contributions, or payment is required for a supposed cure, we must question the cure's effectiveness. A cure is either business or disinterested healing; it cannot be both at the same time. Some might argue that this could be extended to physicians, but this situation is not the same. Doctors have to study hard and keep

---

88   *The Faith Healers* is a 1987 book by magician and skeptic James Randi, with a foreword by Carl Sagan that documents Randi's exploration of the world of faith healing and his exposing the sleight of hand trickery and deceit by its performers.

up with advances in their profession, and they must use equipment and facilities that are expensive and require a supporting staff that has to be paid. Physicians also have a certification or degree that accredits them, and they have experience, which at least guarantees some promising results. Charlatans, on the other hand, formed overnight and appointed as themselves masters, gurus, or healers. They commit one of the worst crimes, which is to exploit the suffering persons.

There is a group that we have not mentioned so far, the indigenous shamans or sorcerers in native autochthonous cultures. These figures served a social function in their community or tribe and formed a hereditary lineage by which knowledge was passed on from father to son or from master to disciples. Their function was not to receive benefits, although they enjoyed prestige. They had real knowledge of the use of plants, minerals, and animals that had some therapeutic properties, knowledge that was achieved after a long series of trials and errors. Time has proved, for example, that herbology's principles are real; in fact, traditional medicine in China continues to successfully apply them. In our Western world, we have incorporated many of the plants' healing principles in drug development. The shamans or sorcerers also possessed rudimentary knowledge of the use of subtle energies, applied usually during rituals or dances or by ingestion of psychotropic substances that induced an altered state of consciousness.

Today many people, using the prestige of these primitive healers, appoint themselves shamans or sorcerers, but they do so purely for commercial purposes. Any of us just by conducting a quick online internet tour search can see how many people offer their tariffed services to patients who are actively and desperately seeking a cure. Again I insist that it is one of the worst crimes to exploit suffering persons. To get in touch with a true shaman, one must penetrate the jungle and locate a member of any of the primitive tribes that still remain on the planet. I do not believe in city shamans or in shaman courses or seminars. It takes almost a lifetime to learn what shamans' ancestors transmitted to them in the form of experience and knowledge.

CHAPTER 15

Qigong Healing

In China we can frequently witness acts of healing conducted by Qigong masters and of course by physicians who practice this technique. Also the television series *Discovery Health* has aired several documentaries showing different treatments with Qigong. On the Internet, especially on YouTube and Dailymotion, one can watch many videos of healing experiences. There are also countless books written on this subject in many languages. But although this practice is already known and widespread, for some people it could be something new. A recent Internet search of the term "Qigong healing" produced about 3,500,000 results. If someone could devote a few minutes just to superficially read the content of this information, it would take at least 11,600 reading hours (nearly four years reading eight hours a day).

I had myself the opportunity to perform several cures that some might describe as miraculous simply because they do not understand the procedures used to control subtle energy. I have performed healing treatments mostly on relatives, close friends, and only in emergencies to strangers. I have refused to become a "healer," since that is the work of physicians; nevertheless, I have had some rewarding experiences in healing by controlling subtle energy with the method of Qigong. But on several occasions, after completing the procedure, I was totally exhausted. When I commented on this situation years later to Master Tian Wu, in Nanjing, he told me that when treating a patient with

Qigong, the healer runs the risk of over-exceeding his capacities, especially for reasons of affections or family ties (when one covets a cure at any cost). In those cases the healer do not just use the universal energy (qi), but he can use some of his own energy. It's like a doctor who, to save a patient, makes a transfusion of his own blood. A better example might be when someone assists someone whose vehicle has a low battery, by connecting in the process depletes his own. This is a very delicate part of therapeutic Qigong (or any other subtle-energy procedure for the same purpose) because by ignorance one can perform an action that, although it improves the patient's health, could harm or exhaust the therapist.

Rosita R.V. was a friend of mine who was suffering from breast cancer with metastasis to the lungs. On several occasions I had done Qigong treatments to improve her quality of life, and she had experienced great improvement that could have been converted into a recession as a side effect. (Treatments with subtle energy for this type of disease are very problematic because they can accelerate the illness process). Only an experienced physician can determine the stage the disease has reached—whether it is in an early stage and can be treated or in an advanced stage, at which point is little or nothing can be done. The same is valid for people with heart troubles, as the treatment with subtle energy accelerates the heart rate. I remember once that Rosita had to undergo chemotherapy but had very low defenses according to hematological tests, so I tried to give her a treatment to boost the immune system. I told her not to say anything about it to her doctor in case that he would be surprised by the sudden increase of lymphocytes T count in the tests. She told him instead that she'd been drinking a tea that her sister had brought from Greece. Later on the doctor kept insisting that she give him a sample of that wonderful and miraculous tea! Later when I had to move out from Miami, where she lived, the treatment was interrupted, and she suffered a decline in her quality of life. Later she returned to Caracas, where I was. Her disease was then at an advanced stage, and she wanted to be with her relatives for her remaining time. On one occasion she called me again, complaining of a severe headache that would not go away with any painkiller, even the strongest. I asked my cousin who is a doctor to accompany me to see her and to examine her heart and lungs. Having determined that she had normal blood pressure, I went forward with the Qigong treatment, and the pain disappeared, to the surprise of my cousin. Unfortunately I found out later on that the pain was due to the pressure from metastasis[89] in her brain, and very little could be done. But surely the Qigong must have released powerful endorphins[90], which fought the sharp pain.

Experiments conducted by Dr. Haruyama[91] and many others have shown that the endorphin known as beta-endorphin is a type of peptide hormone consisting mainly of tyrosine (a kind of amino acid.). The molecular structures of such endorphins, as well as their effects, are very similar to those of the opioid drug morphine. These endorphins activate the human immune system and protect it against degenerative diseases such as cancer. It has been shown that during Qigong treatment, the secretion of these endorphins is increased, which explains its healing effects and especially the pain suppression.

The Liao Fa Qigong can indeed cure many ailments, but its implementation requires medical knowledge (especially that of Chinese acupuncture) as well as extensive experience and practice, so it is easier for Chinese physicians to study Qigong' as a supplementary subject in medical schools. It is usually applied as adjuvant therapy after surgery or trauma because it induces a faster recovery. It has also been used successfully in the treatment of problems related to pregnancy and to speed healing in psychosomatic diseases.

---

89   Metastasis, or metastatic disease, is the spread of a cancer from one organ or part to another nonadjacent organ or part.

90   Endorphins (endogenous morphine) are endogenous opioid peptides that function as neurotransmitters. They are produced by the pituitary gland and the hypothalamus in vertebrates, and they resemble the opiates in their abilities to produce analgesia and a feeling of well-being.

91   See *A Great Revolution in The Brain World*, written by Dr. Haruyama from Tokyo Universty, at http://www.sortlifeout.co.uk.

My most dramatic experience using Qigong therapy was not with humans but with a cat. It is said that cats have nine lives because people see them alive after falling from a great heights. But this is a skill that they have: to turn around and just like people in martial arts, they deflect the force of impact. In this case was not a falling event. Our cat was sleeping under the tire of a jeep from of a visiting friend who, while leaving, backed up his vehicle and partially crushed the poor animal. The cat managed to crawl out, but it had an open wound and an almost macerated abdomen. One of my sons offered to wring its neck to prevent prolonged suffering, but I thought of a better solution—to apply an emergency Qigong treatment. I didn't think it would bring much effect, but it was all I could think to do. It was not possible to sew with stitches the large open wound that would soon become infected. In the following days I applied a few short additional treatments, and against logic and possibilities, the wound, which was not sutured, began to close without infection. After two weeks it was a new cat—even naughtier, in fact. That was a great experience, not just for the healing but because it occurred in the absence of any psychological influence or placebo effect. From that experience, I learned that treatments with subtle energy are effective regardless of the beliefs or mind-set of the treated person.

Laboratory experiments related to Qigong that studied the effects or influence on live animals were carried out at two levels, one at the microscopic level (on bacteria, amoebas, and other unicellular animals) and the other at the macroscopic level (on bigger animals). In some microscopic experiments, Qigong masters have managed to kill colonies of Gram-positive bacteria with the emission of external qi (wei-chi). Regarding treatments on higher animals, significant measured results rule out the influence of suggestion and the placebo effect.

When I personally applied Qigong treatments, usually for relieving pain to postoperative or posttraumatic patients, they totally ignored what Qigong was or meant. I told them that I would provide energy assistance by a special procedure to which they could give any name they wanted, from witchcraft to magic, and that they didn't need to believe in anything to receive its benefits. After brief treatments all said they perceived feelings of pleasant warmth through their bodies. Others reported that they felt lighter, and others just said, "It feels invigorating." I've never treated any person with Qigong who did not as a result feel some kind of sensation, usually pleasant or invigorating. Of course I did not treat too many patients because, as I said, I did not want to be considered a healer. The ones treated were emergency cases or close relatives.

I insist that doctors are the ones trained to know when a more invasive treatment such as surgery is required. In China they use Qigong only when they consider it appropriate, but generally it can be applied during the recovery period and convalescence. I personally do not recommend anyone trying healing without being a doctor. Considering that even doctors themselves can make mistakes, unskilled people are much more likely to commit them; good intentions are not enough. Although an exception can be made in an emergency, even then the patient should seek subsequent professional intervention and a checkup by a physician.

In our Western society we want instant results. We want a pill to make pains disappear immediately; we wish to lay a hand on someone to achieve a miraculous and instantaneous cure. The results of Qigong could be considered miraculous in many cases, but getting to this level requires a lot of time, knowledge, and effort. Currently unscrupulous people in China offer short courses or seminars on Qigong for a few weeks to earn a quick buck. These courses are combined with sightseeing, and they are quite expensive. The worst thing is that these courses are offered to people who are not physicians or related to the medical profession in any way. Grandparents used to describe such situations by comparing them to giving a monkey a razor blade to play. I advise those who like to go sightseeing to do just that. And the doctor who wants to learn therapeutic Qigong can do so in a respectable institution, one that requires at least two years of residency in a hospital, which would be equivalent to a graduate course of study. Further, such a course should be conducted in English; otherwise, it would require many more years during which the student learned Mandarin Chinese.

Overall, Qigong therapy is not something one can learn quickly during a weekend seminar because, as already mentioned, its application requires basic knowledge of anatomy, physiology, and other medical matters. Neophytes should avoid trying to cure a patient without the proper knowledge and training since the patient might suffer irreversible damages. People with medical vocations should study medicine and, if they so desire, complement or increase their knowledge by learning Qigong therapy. Healing is the work of medical doctors who earn a license after studying for many years. Furthermore there is no general healing, just as there is no panacea. A physician should make a specific diagnosis after a rigorous screening. It is appropriate for only advanced Qigong masters to use their knowledge and experience in emergencies or in cases in which traditional medicine has not produced the expected results and there is not a physician available who has knowledge and expertise in Qigong healing.

Being able to manage the subtle energy (qi) with Qigong procedures and then apply it therapeutically means having gone through several stages or levels. The first is the detection and collection of qi. In simpler terms, it is the level at which we become aware of the existence of qi and begin to feel it. It is like putting our fingers to a bare wire to feel the electric shock; until that moment we only knew that there was a circulating electric current (theory), but then we felt its impact (practical verification).

After being in a position to perceive and feel qi, the practitioner can move to a second level where he can accumulate energy, like charging a car battery, or establish an equilibrium in which optimal levels are restored and there is neither excess nor deficiency. The first and second levels are required in almost all variants of Qigong, including martial arts.

The third level is the most complicated, sophisticated, and dangerous, especially in the healing application of Qigong, because at this level one transmits or radiates the internal qi by outwardly emitting it (this irradiated qi is known as *wai-qi*). Just having command of the first two levels does not enable the practitioner to safely actuate in the third one without risks for himself and for the patient.

In China the Qigong Liao Fa for therapeutic purposes is applied in four variants:

1. in combination with traditional Chinese medicine
2. in combination with Western medicine
3. in combination with acupuncture and/or moxibustion
4. alone (only by very advanced masters or doctors)

From a scientific standpoint, the healing or therapeutic Qigong is the best documented and taught, because physicians, having a scientific background, do not accept anything that is not verifiable and repeatable. In China, doctors study Qigong among the subjects in medical schools.

References to Qigong and its procedures date back more than three thousand years. From the Western Zhou dynasty (1100–770 BC), ancient bronze objects contain inscriptions related to Qigong. From the Eastern Zhou dynasty, the principles and training method of Qigong were mentioned on a jade relic. Also found was a painting on silk with forty-four colored illustrations of Daoyin exercises[92] belonging to the first Han dynasty (206–24 BC). Also during the Han dynasty it came into light the first medical treatise, *The Yellow Emperor's Canon of Internal Medicine*,

---

92 Early gymnastic breathing exercises, predecessors of Qigong.

in which systematically the principles of Qigong were established. There are also records about Qigong in the *General Treaty on the Etiology and Symptomatology of the Disease* (610 AD) written by Chao Yanfang during the Sui dynasty[93].

Seeing that more than 3,100 years ago the Chinese already had knowledge of Qigong, it is surprising that Western civilization did not know about it earlier and only rediscovered it in the twentieth century. We do not marvel only at the antiquity of Qigong, but also that of acupuncture. The meridians and acupuncture points, which are centers of energy convergence and used in Qigong therapy, were first described in ancient times. Their use and therapeutic application was transmitted from generation to generation without knowledge of its origins and its scientific basis. Only in the last fifty years, after the invention of the Dermatron[94], could it be scientifically determined that acupuncture points described from ancient times indeed have lower electrical-resistance properties at the skin surface, which clearly differentiates them from the surrounding area. Where did this knowledge come from? It does not correspond with the state of civilization at the time it was first described.

On the origins of this type of knowledge, there are two hypotheses, which I only mention as a reference because their deep analysis is not the object of this book and would require a lengthy discussion. The first hypothesis is that a very advanced civilization already existed, preceding us, and for some cataclysmic reason disappeared, along with many of its achievements. Many ancient documents contain knowledge that we are just rediscovering, and much of it seems to be the legacy of a more advanced civilization. Take, for instance, the writings left by the

---

93   Referred to in *Chinese Qigong*, Publishing House of Shanghai College of Traditional Chinese Medicine, 1990 and 1992.

94   A device to measure the electrical resistance of the skin and other variables, which is used by modern homeopathic physicians. The Dermatron, and its progeny, are basically ohmmeters. Dr. Voll (the inventor) found that over an acupuncture point, there is significantly less skin resistance than over skin in general. Over a normal acupuncture point there is 100,000 ohms of resistance.

ancient sages of India, *rishis*, which were mistakenly interpreted as mere religious texts.

One of the things that surprised me when I studied physics, is that there is a mathematical matrix group known as the Group of Quaternions (Vierkantengruppen) that was described by these rishis in ancient Hindu literature. Later the mathematicians assumed such concept as an abstraction exercise in the science of numbers without any practical application, until it was discovered that subatomic particles movements analyzed in a "heavy water chamber"[95] behaved according to that group of matrix. Could it be possible that an ancient civilization reached levels that we just are approaching and for some reason were lost? Why does the ancient Vedic literature (from India) describe the existence of "winged flying machines" called *vimanas*?

Much new evidence suggests that the Earth might have had periods of major technological advancement. Another of these inexplicable events originates with the Dogon tribe in Mali, West Africa. It is reported that the traditions they narrated for generations demonstrate that they knew about of the existence of the four moons of Jupiter and the rings of Saturn, things that man ignored until the invention of the telescope. They talked about the star Sirius and its unseen companion that rotates every fifty years and is made of a metal that is the heaviest in the universe. Today astronomers have found that there is indeed such a heavenly body, called Sirius-B, but that it can only be detected by supersensitive instruments that the Dogon tribe could not have had. Where did their information come from? In Fritjof Kapra's [96]*The Tao of Physics*, he describes strange similarities between ancient religious writings and recent advances in the sciences, especially physics and astronomy. Our recent ancestors were not able to see these similarities because of their limited progress.

---

95 *Heavy water*, formally called deuterium oxide, or 2H 2O or D2O, is a form of water that contains a larger than normal amount of the hydrogen isotope deuterium (also known as "heavy hydrogen") rather than the common hydrogen-1 isotope that makes up most of the hydrogen in normal water.

96 *The Tao of Physics* by Fritjof Capra, Bantam Books (1980).

The second hypothesis about the origin of this knowledge is the extraterrestrial or alien influence. Some argue that beings from other worlds visited us in the past, leaving us many of these skills. Is Qigong an extraterrestrial legacy? Or is it a legacy from extinct human civilizations? While knowing the origin of this knowledge is interesting, it is not decisive. Whatever it was, human or alien, what is important is that we take advantage of it and do not use it to manipulate our fellow beings.

Cures with Qigong are not like some of the cures depicted in science fiction films, which are often achieved by simply putting hands on the patient. To control and apply Qigong requires different ways of using both the hands and the mind, and most important is that it requires knowledge of anatomy, physiology, and other medical subjects. Especially important is knowledge about the energy or acupuncture points, as Qigong often applies subtle energy focused on those specific points, as is also done with acupressure (applied with fingertips). Finally, the *sine qua non* is the ability to access an altered state of consciousness without rituals or preconditioning.

We should not underestimate this expertise. Here I quote, just as an example, instructions on how to apply Qigong to treat cervical spondylopathy[97]. "*The doctor must first determine which of the four different types it is, whether it is from the nerve root or if it is a myeloid type, if due to vertebral artery or sympathetic nerve*". (How could someone, who is not a doctor, know?). The description continues "*In the last of these types, symptoms include occipital level hemicranias, exophthalmia, brachycardia, etc.*" (What do these terms mean to a layperson?). Once the diagnosis is made based on the previous screening instructions then the treatment could be applied, which I transcribe below and which seems to be reading hieroglyphs: "*Press GB20, apply Wai-Qi (in different ways) in points Du 16, UB10, SI15, SI14, H1, LI 11 LI 4 and Xiaohai SI8 H3*". Isn't that simple? Right?

Subtle-energy management and control for therapeutic purposes can be learned in two ways, the first by trial and error (with consequent

---

97 In medicine, spondylopathy is a general term for disorders of the vertebrae.

health risks for the patient and the practitioner) and the second in medical schools in China or with the guide of a Qigong master versed in medical science. One of the consequences for healers (medical or not) from their possible first successful experiences is beginning to suffer from a syndrome doctors also suffer at some stage early in their career: they feel like they are "playing god" because they naively believe that they could control over life and death. This syndrome quickly disappears with one's first failure or the death of a patient.

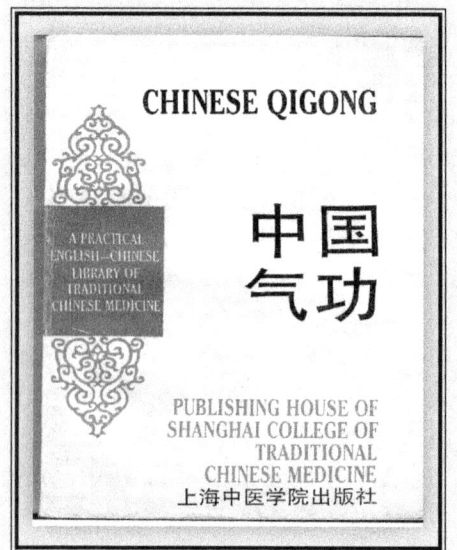

Qigong textbooks at medical level are mostly written in Mandarin Chinese, but I've been fortunate to get some of them to have an English version. The first one is a Chinese-English bilingual edition that is part of a collection of twelve volumes, of which the one on Qigong is the last. The collection has been published by the Publishing House of Shanghai College of Traditional Chinese Medicine.

Another very good and recommended book is *Chinese Qi-gong Therapy*, published by the Shandong Science and Technology Press, which is a compilation of Mr. Zhang Mingwu, director of the National Association for Research on Chinese Qigong, and vice president of the Association for Qigong Research in Beijing. In this latest book he describes five basic patterns for the application of Qigong therapy, followed by the pattern for cancer treatment and the pattern for the treatment of hypertension, massage patterns with application of Qigong, and finally some specific methods to rectify and deviate the treatment. At this time there are many more books being published on this subject in China.

I previously explained that only at the third level of development (that of the external emission of qi or wai qi), can one achieve healing effects. This external qi emission is perceived by both the patient and the practitioner and is an objective sensation free of constraints or suggestions. A patient who ignores the effects or what Qigong really is can be treated without his knowing what he is being submitted to. It's like someone we do not know depositing money in our bank account. Therapeutic Qigong can also be applied from a distance, which sounds fantastic and impossible but has been scientifically demonstrated by Bell's theorem and of course by the results achieved by this practice.

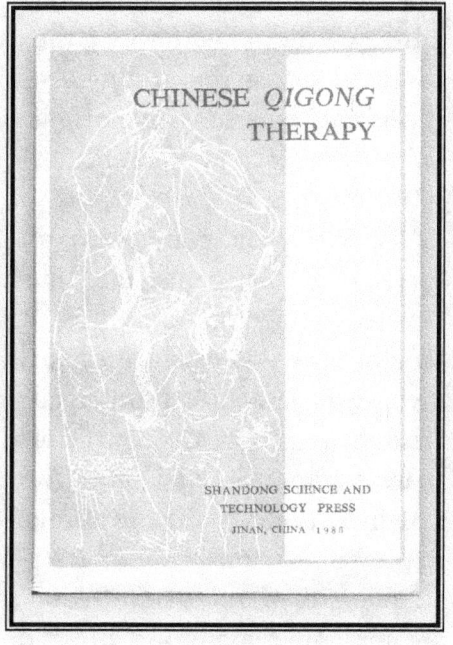

In Qigong therapeutic applications, there are several phenomena or side effects that are perceived as separate sensations by the patient and by the practitioner. When the flow of energy (qi) and irrigation reach a certain point, the practitioner or therapist perceives certain sensations. Among them may be what masters call the "eight touches," which do not occur simultaneously. In fact only one of them may be perceived, depending on the treatment and circumstances. These feelings may be thermal (sensations of heat or cold) or a slight irritation or pain. Or the feelings may be relative to weight (feeling lighter or heavier) or size (feeling larger or smaller). Meanwhile the patient may in turn feel certain sensations during treatment such as heat, cold, vibration, chills, goose bumps, or a sensation of floating or a sinking feeling. The patient may also perceive background lights or sounds. In some reported cases patients have perceived as well a surrounding flower scent (some people named this the fragrance of Qigong).

Part of therapeutic Qigong is applied by means of massage, which may be of four basic types. The first, known as *pu-tong an mo*, is a stress-relief massage to release toxins and improve health. The second type is known as *tui na* and is used to treat minor injuries and certain diseases in addition to significantly improving blood circulation and energy. The third type is applied only on the cavities and is known as *dian xue*. It is also used to treat minor illnesses. The fourth type is the most therapeutic and is applied as curative or adjuvant treatment in many diseases. It is known as *wai qi liao fa*, and its name implies the external emission of subtle energy.

Currently there are many hospitals in China dedicated exclusively to Qigong treatments, and most other hospitals have departments devoted to Qigong. As early as 1955, one of the first modern-era Qigong sanatoriums was established in the city of Tangshan, Hebei Province. Two years later the municipal sanatorium of Qigong in the city of Shanghai was founded. In October 1959 the first national meeting to share experiences of Qigong was held in the city of Beidahe, Hebei Province, under the patronage of the Ministry of Public Health of the Republic of China. About sixty-four units from seventeen provinces attended. It would take too long to list all the medical institutions that are applying Qigong in China, Taiwan, and Singapore, not to mention those established in England, the United States, France, and Germany, among other countries. In 1988 the first World Conference on Medical Research in Qigong took place in the city of Beijing, followed a series of lectures in Tokyo, Berkeley, California,.) and New York. The current offer on courses, books, and videos about medical Qigong is extensive.

Medicine has become so complicated that there are now countless specialties and sub specialties. It is not uncommon that a patient be treated or examined simultaneously by two or three specialists, which means that doctors recognize their own limitations in certain areas and call their colleagues to interdisciplinary cooperate in solving a problem.

Likewise, the therapeutic application of Qigong is not a universal panacea that cures all. We must recognize that it is very useful and produces surprising results in a number of conditions, and its effectiveness is even greater when combined with traditional Chinese medicine, acupuncture, or Western medicine.

Qigong medical applications, taking into account the above caveats, require the ability to release qi (or, also, *convey* qi), which is not as easy as it seems. In either of the two variants, healers should avoid using their own qi and transferring it to others; it is instead a simultaneous process of capture and emission of qi. The success of Qigong masters is to transfer external captured qi and not use his own accumulated qi. In these cases the practitioner serves only as a means (or transducer) that connects the external qi with the person who requires it, either to create balance or compensate for a deficiency. Neophytes, who mostly ignore this process, could intend to heal others but end up making use of their own qi, which, if significantly reduced, would result in physical disorders and mental fatigue.

"The Chinese Health Qigong Association" was established in 2000 as a government agency to regulate public Qigong practice, restricting the number of people that could gather at a time, requiring state-approved training and certification of instructors, limiting practice to four standardized forms of daoyin from the classical medical tradition, and encouraging other types of recreation and exercise such as yoga and tai chi.

CHAPTER 16

Superstrength and
Martial Arts

Most Chinese words came to the West with the first emigrants, who were from Canton (Guangzhou), a province in the south of China where the language, Cantonese, had also been the language used in Hong Kong, which was a British colony until 1999. Most contacts and business abroad, especially during the Cold War era, were made via Hong Kong and by Cantonese immigrants who spoke the same language. Westerners thus came to know Chinese martial arts as *kung fu*, which is basically an expression in the Cantonese language; likewise, we used to call Beijing, China's capital, *Peking*. The large number of Cantonese who immigrated to the United States for the construction of railways, especially in the state of California, were treated rudely. Many of their customs—such as carrying palanquins—were banned to keep them from being assimilated into the society, and these limitations forced them to live in ghettos known today as Chinatowns. They had difficulty communicating with others, mainly because the Cantonese language is complicated, and only they could understand themselves.

California residents at the time were surprised to see how the small-statured Chinese sometimes defeated bigger people in fights or struggles. It is said that when the Westerners asked the Chinese about these combat techniques and the Chinese tried to explain that they were not easy to learn, their explanation was that they required "much time and effort," or in Cantonese, they required "kung fu." This description, which applies to *any* activity or learning that takes time and effort became the American term for the Chinese practice when listeners misheard or misinterpreted the explanation. In the Mandarin language (now the official language) the term to refer to the martial art is *wu shu*, which means "art of war," and now both terms are used in the West to refer to Chinese martial arts.

The origin of Chinese fighting techniques and martial arts is lost in time, and many stories are confusing. There's no doubt that during the advance of civilization, specialized groups for combat were established, and the role of soldiers was created. This required techniques of attack and defense, and so training for such emerged. People realized that during times of peace they also had to be prepared for war and not treat it like something unexpected or unusual, especially if the lack of preparation and the surprise element had previously caused them heavy losses.

Through observation, as well as by trial and error, they perfected their techniques, and they incorporated some strategies from their ordinary life. Among the everyday experiences that were most useful for combat was a technique used in subsistence hunting—mentally focusing on a target. They also noticed that in combat the peasants who were more robust withstood the battle in better condition and survived the most; hence physical strengthening exercises were introduced.

Later in the Taoist monasteries falconry and archery were developed, for which concentration was paramount. At that time the formula for success was established. It consisted of a combination of mental focus on a target with strengthening body exercises. The higher the concentration and physical preparation, the better the combatants were able to perform. But one could not go without the other. Being very strong and well-armed (with sword or spear) had little value because at any distraction or loss of concentration, a soldier could suffer injury or death. From this one of the basic principles of Qi-Gong was established, the mind-body interaction that is achieved by great concentration.

A scroll from the Han dynasty (202 BC) contains martial and therapeutic techniques with symbolic gestures that seem magical and sacred. The first type of combat was performed with bare hands, and the technique—which became famous—was known as *chuan-shu*. Taoism exerted a great influence on the use of this technique by creating special schools for its teaching. A famous Taoist physician, Hua Tuo (220 BC), observed the behavior of various animals and developed an exercise method based on the top five animals, five being at that time the same quantity of elements in their alchemy.

It has been reported that troops used the *wu shu* during the reign of the Yellow Emperor (Tchon Tchi Won), who is said to have ordered the destruction of all documents and chronicles, which made it difficult to confirm historical accuracy. Buddhists meanwhile were alleging that a *bodhisattva* [98] (bo-dhi-dharma) with the name of Po-Ti-Tamo, who was the first patriarch of Chinese Buddhism, introduced in Cathay (China) the ancient martial art from India and taught it, along with his religious beliefs, in a monastery that eventually has become a symbol of Chinese martial arts and is known as the Shaolin temple[99].

There he began to spread Buddhist practices to a group of novices, also teaching them the execution of twelve moves and twenty-four muscle exercises called *ichin-ching*. With these one could acquire a remarkable physical body and a great ability to concentrate. When the monks began training with these exercises in their morning practices, they acquired very strong bodies. These movements were based on natural movements that replicated the forms of twelve kinds of different animals.

Kung fu or wushu is seen by many of its supporters as a guide to spiritual development rather than as a self-defense technique. Martial arts grouped under the above terms have been strongly influenced by

---

98   According to Tibetan Buddhism, a bodhisattva is one of the four sublime states a human can achieve in life (the others being an arhat, Buddha, or pratyekabuddha). In general in Buddhism, a bodhisattva is an enlightenment (*bodhi*) being (*sattva*).

99   In the Shaoshi Mountains some 13 km northwest of Defeng, under the peak of Wuru is the Shaolin Temple. Its name comes from being located in the woods just north of Mount Shaolin, Henan Province.

Confucianism, Taoism, and Buddhism. The kung Fu or Wushu from Shaolin temple is one of the oldest and most respected martial arts in the world. It evolved over more than fifteen hundred years, giving rise to many systems, not just Chinese (such as *wing chun* and *hung gar*) but also Japanese (such as Shorinji Kenpo). It was said that one Shaolin monk was worth a thousand soldiers. The techniques supposedly originated in the Shaolin temple are grouped as *Shao-Lin-Quan*.

In a show of the Beijing Chinese Circus that was touring our city, performers were beaten with sharp axes in the chest, then with swords, and then they were firmly pressed in the throat with spearheads. They broke solid bricks with their fists and performed many wonders of super force and superstrength. This is the type of Qigong applied to martial arts to obtain superstrength.

I have a recorded documentary about Qigong filmed in Malaysia, where one can see unusual human actions, like jumping from a three-story building and falling on hard concrete floor, jumping from even higher places and falling on grass, jumping through glass walls to lower levels, and jumping from cars moving at high speeds. All these extreme actions did not cause any harm to the performers (except minor cuts when they crossed through the glass walls). In another event masters present there poured boiling oil first on a plant, which was burned or fried completely, and then on people, who did not suffer the slightest burn; only their skin showed a reddening. Also filmed was the training received by children under eight—adults hit them in the chest with the fist without their feeling or showing any pain. Then some women were hit hard with wooden clubs on their backs, and they remained unmoved. To conclude, one of the masters was buried alive for three days and survived.

In short, the Qigong applied to martial arts is a mixture of knowledge and skill. First of all, a physical strengthening is required, which is achieved by a combination of exercises accompanied by mental interaction. Thereafter one should go through concentration drills, and finally he or she should acquire knowledge of acupuncture and anatomy. All these are like the ingredients of a recipe: if one is missing or if the procedure of preparation is not followed correctly, it will not be possible to get the expected results.

CHAPTER 17

Psychic Applications and Exceptional Human Functions

So far we have distinguished various types of Qigong with different applications or objectives. For many the most interesting, and in turn the most mysterious, is the one dealing with generating, develop and increasing paranormal psychic abilities, also known as *exceptional human functions* (telepathy, clairvoyance, premonitions, clairaudience, telekinesis, remote viewing, and so on). This type of Qigong spawned countless myths and legends that were only recently been considered as to have a certain level of credibility based on the latest scientific research. These unique capabilities within Qigong were developed mostly in monasteries, while therapeutic or healing Qigong flourished outside.

In relation to this, it is important to stress the fact that I'm not trying to sell any particular idea, so I am not obliged to highlight the advantages or hide the disadvantages of Qigong; neither am I introducing something based on half-truths. Rather, what follows is a fairly simple analysis that can provide guidance for others. It is based on my personal experience and complemented by research on the latest developments in this field as well as those of the new physics.

Let's also make clear what the terms *abnormal, paranormal,* or *extrasensory* really mean. Formerly a division was created (artificial for many), between those perceptions so far considered normal, and the so-called paranormal, extra-sensory, or psychic phenomena. In 1942 Robert Thouless, a British psychologist, introduced the word *psi* to refer to psychic phenomena, but this just added to the confusion, especially in several foreign languages, because it is considered just a prefix, so the rest of the word seems to be missing part of expression. In short, everything that was not perceived by our traditional five senses fell under the heading of paranormal. In the meantime a new term was coined— *exceptional human functions* (EHF).

Although these capacities are considered extraordinary or paranormal, they are something that we are experience nearly every day, just as we do with our "normal" capacities. The different levels we can observe in normal physical capacities (athletic endeavors) and mental capacities (music, performing arts, and poetry, among others) make us infer that there are different levels as well in people who have "abnormal" capacities. But in any case, those inborn EHF capacities could be enhanced in the same way people enhance their other capacities—by studying or training (the way athletes, musicians, or artists do).

By accepting the term *exceptional human functions*, we acknowledge as well that these are indeed human functions, and that these are not normal but exceptional abilities. This means that not everybody will make use of them, and even those who do will not do so at all times. The good news is that it has been proven that these are inborn characteristics that all of us have and that they could be enhanced and used not only exceptionally but purposely.

When the expression *extra sensory perception* was created, scholars wanted to include in that group all signals received by the brain through channels different from our traditional senses. For example, a dream in which we see a scene as it were a movie would be an extra sensory perception because the normal channel for receiving images is through our eyes, photo-receptor sense, and the image in the dream did not originate or depart from those receptors.

The following experiences, among others, are nowadays considered as extrasensory perceptions: *telepathy* (reception and transmission of thoughts); *clairvoyance* (perception of events or images in remote time and space); *remote vision,* (a type of clairvoyance that allows one to get images or events in real time from faraway locations); *premonitions* (anticipated knowledge of something about to happen); *retro cognition* (access to events remote in time and space that have already occurred); *clairaudience* (perception of sounds or spoken language remote in time and space); and *telekinesis* (moving physical objects or making changes thereof). Some people include in this group *lucid dreams* (conscious interactions in the normal dreams) as well as those feelings of attraction or repulsion to certain people or places. Later in this chapter all these capacities will be discussed in detail.

These phenomena are more common and widespread than many persons think or have been aware of, a fact that is confirmed by the worldwide flow of information among many cultures and nationalities. Institutions that began investigating these phenomena more than thirty or forty years ago created a new branch of psychology called *parapsychology.* The files and databases of these institutions are full of cases that have been extensively verified and documented. Their research is now focused more on the causes for these behaviors than their existence. In regard to the mechanisms that produce these phenomena, several theories have been proposed, some linked to infrared radiation, others to electromagnetism, and others to subatomic events. Other schools are aimed at exposing what we have always considered our reality and taking us into a quantum world where multiple realities coincide simultaneously. There are two important theories worthy of being discussed and analyzed, the theory of entanglement[100] or

---

100   Also known as quantum entanglement, which is a quantum mechanical phenomenon in which the quantum states of two or more objects have to be described with reference to each other, even though the individual objects may be spatially separated. Quantum entanglement has applications in the emerging technologies of quantum computing and quantum cryptography and has been used to realize quantum teleportation experimentally.

interconnectedness and Bell's Theorem[101], but due to their complexity, they are beyond the scope of this book.

The first serious papers on extrasensory phenomena, not accepted at that time, occupied more than eleven thousand pages between 1882 and 1900 in *Proceedings and Journal of the Society for Physical Research* in London. Early those scientists who were permeated by mechanistic physics refused to accept these phenomena of the mind, so in 1876 when Sir William Barrett spoke of his experimental work on telepathy before the British Association for the Advancement of Science, he was mocked by the participants, and the Association refused to publish his paper.

Going back in history, the paranormal psychic powers or capacities that come with the practice of Qigong are similar to the powers known as siddhis in raja-yoga. These powers are fully described also in the *Yoga Sutras* of Patanjali. In ancient times many of these phenomena were reported in many cultures and attributed to saints, oracles, prophets, Sufis, sorcerers, seers, shamans, and sages. Many of these phenomena could not be explained by the knowledge at that time and were so regarded as miraculous.

In esoteric Islam (Sufis), powers linked to altered states of consciousness are mentioned like those known in India as siddhis, which could be obtained at the level of *shahood* (Arabic: دوهش, "evidence"). At this level a person can get any information about any event or person with his will. This stage is broadly categorized according to activation of the senses: the person can see things anywhere in the universe (remote

---

101 What makes Bell's theorem unique and powerful is that it shows that nature violates the most general assumptions behind classical pictures, not just details of some particular models. No combination of local deterministic and local random variables can reproduce the phenomena predicted by quantum mechanics and repeatedly observed in experiments. The title of Bell's Theorem is based in his seminal article that challenged the completeness of quantum mechanics. In his paper, Bell started from the same two assumptions as did Einstein, Podolsky and Rosen, namely (1) reality (that microscopic objects have real properties determining the outcomes of quantum mechanical measurements), and (2) locality (that reality in one location is not influenced by measurements performed simultaneously at a distant location). Bell was able to derive from those two assumptions an important result, namely Bell's inequality, implying that at least one of the assumptions must be false. What is powerful about Bell's theorem is that it doesn't refer to any particular physical theory..

vision or clairvoyance) and hear things anywhere in the universe (clairaudience). The person can smell things anywhere in the universe and touch things anywhere in the universe as well. Sufis also define a state called *fatah* (Arabic: حتف, "opening, victory") present at the peak of *shahood*. At this stage, the person doesn't need to close his eyes for meditation. He or she is freed from both space and time. According to their teachings, the person can see, hear, taste, and touch anything that is present anywhere in time and space.

At first, when psychic abilities levels are increased by either the practice of Qigong, or any other esoteric method, terrible dilemma is presented to us, one that is very difficult to elucidate or clarify. Because we previously desired that some facts or events be accomplished, when they in fact come to be, we cannot know whether we produced them ourselves (due to the preliminary desire) or whether we had a premonition. At that point, people become very cautious with their thoughts and try to avoid associating desires with them. Believe me, it's really a terrible feeling, like playing with fire and not knowing if you're going to burn yourself, burn others, or set fire to everything around you.

The acquisition of such powers with the practice of Qigong are based on a simple recipe that requires three ingredients: (1) concentrated attention, (2) expression of an intention, and (3) empowerment through access to an altered state of consciousness. To say that the recipe is simple does not mean one should expect immediate outcomes. Long, strict, and hard training are required. Like all recipes, it also carries an implicit warning about what should not be done and what precautions need to be taken.

The first paranormal ability that is developed with Qigong exercises, whether people like it or not, is intuition (anomalous cognition), though it is often not considered a paranormal capacity. This development derives from the balance achieved between the two hemispheres of the brain. To male humans, this development of intuition is more noticeable, although not greater than the one our female counterparts are naturally endowed with.

Parallel to the development of intuition comes the awakening of *telepathy* and similar paranormal capacities, *clairvoyance* and *clairaudience*. These developments are present from the first practice, which is like peeking through a window to what can be achieved later, whatever the primary objective could be.

In the expansion of psychic capacities the development of **psychokinetic** powers follows, which refers to the action of the mind over physical objects (moving, breaking, or altering them). Some people report as well an increased capacity by which one could materialize, transport, or make physical objects disappear, actions that seem magical or impossible, but are worth being considered and studied.

This type of Qigong involves three controversial aspects. The first aspect refers to the innate ability of humans to access and to act on a different mental level, which many people have called exceptional, paranormal, extrasensory, or metaphysical (which is an altered state of consciousness). The second aspect is the capacity to immediately access that altered state of consciousness without the help of rituals or conditioning of any kind, which allows the manipulation of universal energy (qi) to act on material objects and people. The third aspect is the ability to make or produce paranormal phenomena at will by a manifested and enhanced intention at the level of the control element (psyche, mind, or spirit).

The exceptional or paranormal effects resulting from the practice of Qigong are the same effects observed in other cultures and procedures when humans gain access to an altered state of consciousness. Let's be clear: Qigong is the name given to a science whose objective is the manipulation of universal energy known to the Chinese as qi, but it is the same energy that has been controlled and used in different cultures and under different procedures, and all of them have achieved more or less similar outcomes. The big difference is that the Qigong does not make use of rituals, dogmas, group affiliation, or instruments or external reinforcements (optical, sonic, or chemical conditioning).

By using an example from our daily life, we can better understand the above. Let's suppose we want to move from one city to another. This can be accomplished by walking, riding a horse, cycling or traveling in a motor vehicle. The goal, which is to get to the other city, will be achieved regardless of the transportation means; the difference is the required time and effort. Qigong would be the equivalent to the motor vehicle—the fastest way. In addition to being faster, it is also more comfortable because it does not require conditionings such as music, lights, rituals, or chemicals.

It is the only method that accepts the phenomena from a scientific point of view and it does not intend to use the results to attract followers or worshipers, neither for campaign purposes nor to obtain monetary gains. On the contrary, what it does is expose the falsehood of all those beliefs, religions, or groups that claim that these phenomena are linked to a particular school of thought or certain religious or pagan practices.

The phenomena that are produced by Qigong, to which we referred above as extrasensory or paranormal, have been studied for more than thirty years by researchers who are engaged in a specialty called *psychotronics*. This new science is the next stage of investigation, which comes after verifying that the phenomena really exist. It analyzes the hidden causes or origins of the paranormal phenomena and events resulting from controlling vital energy (qi) and tries to define or clarify them in scientific terms.

The Czech mathematician and physicist Julius Krmessky[102] calculated the force required to make a blade turn at 1.2 x 10E-3 dynes and introduced the concept of *psychotronics power*, which is the personal term he used to describe the energy qi. He reported the following:

> *"There is no heat or air radiation, the emission of this energy goes through the glass, water, wood, paper, all metals, even iron and its strength is not diminished by this, and it seems that the human mind can control it."*

---

102 Dr. Julius Krmessky, an outstanding Czech mathematician and physicist, tackled this unexplained energy radiating from humans and published an important scientific paper for the Chair of Physics of the Pedagogical Institute of Trnava.

These facts have been explained as well by Bell's Theorem[103] which explains the existence of a "nonlocal world" in which changes can be transmitted in unusual ways. According to this theorem, these changes are not manipulated or restricted and are immediate or "more than immediate" when transmission anticipates the event. Nick Herbert says that this connection or link between points A and B in the nonlocal world are not subject to any interference between the connected parts. Nothing crosses their space, so no physical matter can hinder this interaction. Its power is neither reduced nor attenuated, as happens, for instance, to radio or television broadcasts (which become weaker with increasing distance). These nonlocal influences are equally powerful a millimeter away as a million miles away. Furthermore they are immediate. The transmission speed is not limited to the speed of light, so a nonlocal connection is established without crossing any space, without attenuation, and without delay, meaning it is not interfered, not attenuated, and immediate.

This modern scientific theory, still in an experimental stage, has much in common with the scientific knowledge of the ancient Indian sages (rishis) who referred to the same phenomena, although with other terms. For them, this nonlocal and non-temporal world dimension was known as *para-atman* which translates as "super ego" or "superior self," perhaps similar to Jung's concept of the *collective unconscious*[104], the *noosphere*[105]of Teylhard de Chardin, the Greek *Logos* of Philo, or *Abzu*, the "sea of knowledge"[106]of the ancient Sumerians. In quantum physics it is a matter of another dimension (s). Rupert Sheldrake in his book

---

103   See the book *Quantum Reality* by Nick Herbert (New York: Anchor Books, 1987).

104   The Swiss psychiatrist Carl. G. Jung, called "the father of transpersonal psychology," suggested the existence of a "collective unconscious"—a deep level of consciousness that is shared by all humans and that seems to transcend time and space.

105   For Teylhard, the noosphere emerges through and is constituted by the interaction of human minds. The noosphere has grown in step with the organization of the human mass in relation to itself as it populates the Earth. As humankind organizes itself in more complex social networks, the higher the noosphere will grow in awareness.

106   *Abzu* in Sumerian means "sea of knowledge," but also "gate" or "portal of wisdom."

Morphic Resonance: The Nature of Formative Causation[107] attributes these phenomena to "entangled particles" in a *morphic resonance field*. This entanglement concept, also known as quantum nonlocality or quantum nonseparability, comes from quantum physics and was mentioned by Albert Einstein as "spooky action at a distance."

Individuals who are not prepared or properly guided by an instructor to experience those newly enhanced powers tend to become infatuated, exhibiting excessive and ridiculous self-satisfaction. They become pedantic, conceited, or arrogant believing, they are supermen or superwomen, placed well above the rest of us. They call themselves masters or gurus and seek to exercise power or control over those around them. But eventually that feeling will produce mental imbalances and frustration when they see their powers disappear or become aware of the limitations of the same in accordance with the objectives and applications. But now let's analyze the exceptional human functions in detail.

Intuition (Anomalous Cognition)

Hunches or intuitions are those experiences in which one has a feeling of knowing or perceiving something in advance about a situation, person, or incident. This experiences do not involve communication with words, and the recipient does not know where this knowledge comes from. But what is intuition? Some consider it an intimate and instantaneous perception of an idea or a truth that becomes evident to those who have it. Who hasn't known exactly what he or she had to do in a situation even though one does not know where the hints were coming from. Who has not had the sense that he knew what was going to happen—and then it did? Many people define intuition as the perception of information through nonphysical senses. It is also known as the sixth sense, feminine instinct, and other terms. In short, it is the direct perception of something existing that is shown in an immediate

---

107 *Morphic Resonance* by Rupert Sheldrake (Park Street Press, 2009).

and concrete way (i.e., without the intervention of other knowledge). It is alleged that intuition is a mechanism for access to the unconscious and by extension to the collective unconscious.

The *Merriam-Webster* dictionary list three meanings for *intuition*: a natural ability or power that makes it possible to know something without any proof or evidence; a feeling that guides a person to act a certain way without fully understanding why; or something that is known or understood without proof or evidence.

Paradoxically all of us know the exact or approximate meaning of the word, and yet in most psychology books references to it are mostly avoided. Some even say that scientists flee in terror when they hear it.

Since our childhood we have heard praise and acclaim for so-called women's intuition. At times many of us males felt handicapped because the females of our species had a tool for life that we didn't. Being "rational men" definitely puts us at a disadvantage with the intuitive sex.

A friend of mine who is a psychiatrist said that we should pay more attention to intuition than reason. Many people were saved from serious accidents or dangerous situations by paying attention to their own intuition, which seems to function as a primitive defense mechanism. Grandparents used to advise youth, "Heed your intuition." Intuitive impulses to proceed with, or suppress a particular action are very strong and difficult to define. It rather appears that we knew that something was right or wrong without knowing the reason or motive, nor whence the information came from.

The elders said that intuition was linked to the heart (feeling) and not to the head (reason). In fact, when we have a hunch or intuition, often it is contrary to reason. All of us have at some point made a decision based on our intuition, and even though at that moment it was neither logical nor appropriate, nevertheless it produced a favorable outcome. For instance, we may, based on a hunch, change our route home, taking a detour for no apparent reason, only to find out that our usually journeyed street was blocked by an accident. How did we have access to the information that the street we use every day was blocked that time? Roulette players tend to follow their intuition, and it seems to help them win, even against the odds. Many successful entrepreneurs attribute their triumphs to having relied more on intuition than reason when making a decision. Some books deeply study these processes of making business decisions guided by intuition; among others we recall *The Logic of Intuitive Decision Making*[108] and *The Role of Intuition in Leadership*[109] authored by Dr. Weston Argor, who reports a case in a cosmetic company where someone made the following comment: "An executive with a PhD from Harvard would be lost here, as we make most of our decisions based on intuition."

A former police investigator told me that a large percentage of crimes are solved using intuition. He says, "A good cop should know how to follow hunches." Police officers' intuition is sometimes linked with the process called retro cognition (a certain type of clairvoyance), which allows them to obtain information on hidden events that have already occurred. Many people call officers with this capacity "police bloodhounds."

Practicing Qigong gives the males of the species the opportunity to catch up with their female counterparts and even surpass them. Every time we make use of this newly enhanced tool that we previously did not have, we will be surprised and astonished, and likely we will regret not having been aware of its advantages. The problem for males, in particular, then, is to separate our rational thought process from the intuitive insights.

Telepathy

After the First World War (1914–1918), the scientific community experienced a resurgence of interest in telepathic phenomena and premonitory dreams. Striking were the many reported cases of soldiers' relatives who perceived the death or serious injury of their loved ones at

---

108 *The Logic of Intuitive Decision Making* by Weston Agor (Greenwood Press, 1986).
109 *The Role of Intuition in Leadership* by Weston Agor (Sage Publications, 1989).

exactly the time that such an event occurred, despite the great distance between them. This type of large-scale recounting of similar telepathic experiences was repeated during the Second World War (1939–1945) and the Vietnam War (1955–1975).

One of the most intriguing and studied phenomenon in the recent past was telepathy. Human beings have for years been in search of the origin of premonitory events and prophecies. Telepathy is often defined as a mind-to-mind connection. In 1882 the Society for Psychical Research in London studied this phenomenon and published in 1886 a

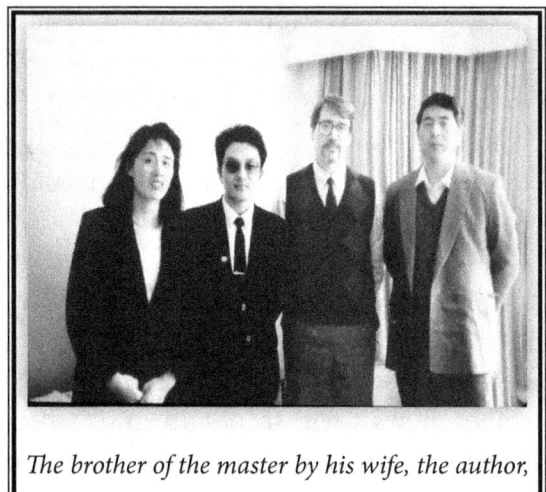

The brother of the master by his wife, the author, and a journalist of Xin Hua

work in two volumes authored by Gurney, Myers, and Podmore. They reported at least seven hundred well-documented cases about telepathic communications. At that time people were doubtful about the existence of telepathy even though they believed in prophets, seers, and the like.

During a visit to Beijing (Peking), the brother of Qigong Master Chang Linfen and his wife were kind enough to take me to a Buddhist temple where a monk with extraordinary psychic (extrasensory) ability happened to live. Profiting from that opportunity, I tried to ask him some questions. The monk seemed the personification of the seated Buddha, with a plump texture, a smooth and radiant face, and a smile always on his lips. Add to this his environment—a beautiful living room with many ancient wood carvings in which he sat on large silk cushions—all of which created the impression of a painting or a film of ancient China.

My Chinese language skills are very limited, so I communicated mainly in English. The monk spoke only his native language, so we had to rely on our friends (the master's brother and his wife) as interpreters. At one point during our exchange, I became frustrated because I realized, from the inconsistent responses of the monk, that the translation was not being properly made and that my friends had only a limited knowledge of English.

It struck me as a solution to ask my translator and the monk (by making use of gestures) to conduct a meditation together, to which the monk agreed. He invited me to take a cushion and sit at his feet in front of him. Once in a meditative state (altered state of consciousness) I intended to convey to the monk my concerns, which were previously expressed verbally and had not been properly answered due to misunderstanding.

To my great surprise, he immediately established a telepathic connection that resembled being connected online to a search engine. The monk gave me answers to all the things I had wanted to ask him, communicating them in the form of 'packages similar to those transmitted in computers. He sent me all the information in a block that could be opened later on individually as files. That transmission time must have been just a few milliseconds, and it definitely was not a verbal communication. Accessible answers and knowledge I never have had before suddenly popped up in my mind.

The experience I just described is similar to the states of "ecstasy with knowledge" or "revelation," in which the person during an altered state of consciousness (ecstasy or trance) acquires knowledge that he did not have before, but he does not know the source or origin.[110] It is also similar to intuition, which is based on knowledge that we take for granted without knowing its origin. Undoubtedly, this experienced monk had had the opportunity for many years to exercise and increase his extrasensory powers. This is just an example of the exceptional or paranormal capabilities a human being can develop when he is devoted to increasing them.

Every day we experience telepathic event and most of the time we are not paying attention to them or we are unaware of them. Telepathic experiences include intuitive hunches, good or bad feelings toward parties so far unknown to us, and the sense of being stared at. To most of us it has

---

110   Stace, W. T. *The Teachings of the Mystics.* New York: New American Library, 1960.

happened more than once that our phone is about to ring or is ringing already, and we perceive who the caller is, even if it's who doesn't call us regularly. In a lab experiment, Doctors Rupert Sheldrake and Pamela Smart[111]conducted trials on this type of experience. They designated four participants who were to identify who was calling them before picking up the receiver. In each of the tests, the participants had four different potential options, and the experimenter selected one at random. They were videotaped and timed during the process. When the phone started ringing, the participants were to tell the camera who was calling and where that person could probably be located. In some cases they even added a comment regarding their level of sureness about each chosen option. The calling parties were some miles far away and in some instances thousands of miles away. The random possibilities to guess who the caller was were around 25 percent, but in a total of 271 trials, there were 122 correct choices, which equals 45 percent, far above the random chances.

The existence of premonitory dreams seems to be one type of telepathy if we understand this as a nonconventional way to receive information in our brain without using the normal senses (sight, smell, taste, touch, and hear). In the dream laboratory at the Maimonides Medical Center in Brooklyn, New York, some interesting experiments were conducted that link telepathy to dreams. (In this context, it is not the same to be asleep as to be dreaming.) In one of these experiments, researchers placed a person in an isolated compartment where the physiological reactions could be monitored while the person was asleep. In the moment the person started to have dreams (a stage detected by rapid eyes movement), a second person outside the cubicle was instructed to act as a telepathic transmitter of certain images. Researcher hoped to find what percentage, if any, of the images dreamt by the person were influenced by the person that telepathically transmitted them. Untimately these experiments were not able to detect any anomaly in the increasing of brain waves, electric signals, or any other response, so the mechanisms of telepathy remain

---

111   See *Journal of Parapsychology*, "Videotaped Experiments on Telephone Telepathy" (Spring 2003) by Rupert Sheldrake and Pamela Smart.

unknown. The Bell theorem mentioned before seems to be the only explanation that provides solutions and clarifications in this matter.

These human capacities such as telepathy enable us as well to conduct the so-called interspecies communication—communicating with animals and plants without the use of spoken language. We have always thought that conversation is a sign of intelligence, but many scientists argue that conversation is just a simple code of communication between humans and that the other species have other forms of communications. Based on this fact, there cannot be a sufficiently rich communication channel between different species, but lately a specialty has emerged that has been termed *interspecies telepathy*[112], a nonverbal but mental form of communication with other species. Nowadays one can find in some countries persons specialized in this technique who proclaim they are interspecies communicators[113]. Some people are indeed able to conduct such communications at the experimental and scientific level, but we have to recognize fraudulent cases of people who offer their services to wealthy owners of pets in order to supposedly transmit to them the alleged concerns of the animals. Of course, those pets have no way to refute or contravene what was told by the communicator.

This actually is not a new discovery but a verification of something we've all experienced in one way or another. Anyone who has had a pet has likely realized that some form of communication with them exists. Many details on this topic are available in the book *The Gift of Interspecies Communication*.[114]

There are many scientific studies that demonstrate that telepathic communications are not only human but have been observed in other animal species and even plants. *The Psychic Power of Animals*[115] reports on an experiment conducted by Pierre Duval and Evelyn Montredon[116] in

---

112 http://www.cyberark.com

113 Interspecies communication is a field of considerable debate, as there is no concrete definition of what constitutes communication.

114 *The Gift of Interspecies Communication* by Nancy Orlen Weber, Unlimited Mind Communications Inc.

115 Schul, Bill. *The Psychic Power of Animals*. New York: Fawcett, 1977.

116 "ESP Experiments with Mice." (1968). Duval, Pierre and Montredon, Evelyn, in *Journal of Parapsychology*, 32(3), 153-166. There are reports that these names were pseudonyms.

France. In this experiment hamsters and gerbils were placed in a box divided into two parts by a partition that allowed a relatively low jump from to either side. A metal plate was placed in each of the two sections that produced an electric shock at intervals chosen at random by an electronic device. In a significant number of events, it was demonstrated that the animals seemed to know in advance on which side the discharge would take place, and when this happened, they were already on the other side. As the intervals were not regular but were generated at random, there was no possible way for the animals to schedule their positions, so it is considered that the animals had the ability to foresee the event, or glimpse their immediate future.

Dr. Rupert Sheldrake[117] wrote a book entitled *Dogs That Know When Their Owners Are Coming Home and Other Unexplained Powers of Animals*. Sheldrake ruled out such factors as smells, sounds, or time of day. He also reported dogs that prevented that their owners commit suicide, as if they knew in advance of their master's intentions. The book includes reports of abnormal animal behavior before earthquakes and other disturbances, all of which can only be explained by some kind of telepathic communication between animals and their owners.

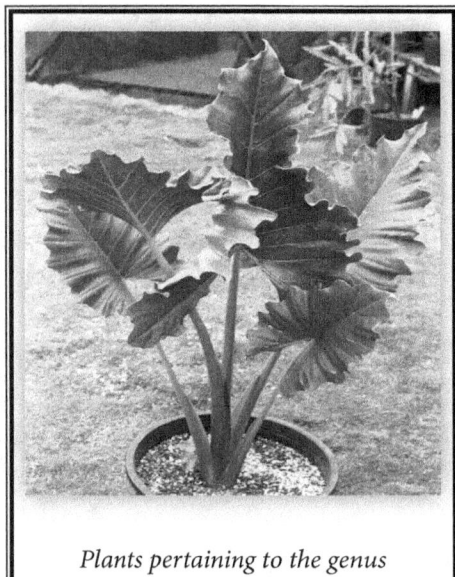

Plants pertaining to the genus Philodendron

As for plants, a reputed Japanese researcher, Dr. Ken Hashimoto,[118] managed to connect very sensitive electrodes to a cactus plant and was thus able to measure reactions that virtually allowed teaching the plant to

117 Go the link www.sheldrake.org.
118 Le Double Langage des Végétaux En l'autre monde Avril 1992 No. 129 Paris. Pp 58–60.

count up to twenty. Another researcher, Dr. Cleve Backster,[119] measured the reactions in a plant of the genus philodendron through electrodes similar to those used in lie detectors and saw how it reacted to a human who supposedly "intended to burn the plant." He was surprised to find that the plant was able to grasp the threat telepathically. In another reported experiment by Paul Savin, he connected to a philodendron plant some sensitive electrodes that were in turn fixed to a trigger mechanism of a garage door. When he was approaching home, the scientist sent a telepathic signal to the plant announcing his arrival; the plant got his command, and its reaction was detected by the electrodes, which in turn induced the garage door to open so he could park his vehicle.

There are many case studies of plants, especially of the genus philodendron, that react to human thought. The reaction of plants to certain music has been conclusively demonstrated, and we know that the Kirlian effect was discovered through experiments that allowed plants to capture the energy field around them.

There are many reported cases of spontaneous or scheduled events in which animals or humans breached through the time barrier of the present time. But it is possible to cross not only the barrier of time but also that of space. In one experiment a boxer dog was locked inside a hermetically isolated, soundproof room and connected to electrocardiograph electrodes. Outside its female owner was submitted to an untimely surprise by a man who attacked her verbally. The dog immediately showed a cardiac reaction when its owner was attacked, despite the attack's being out of his auditory, olfactory, and visual range.

In this era of dominance of the experimental sciences, it has been endlessly shown that telepathy is a natural human ability that is verifiable and quantifiable. It has been studied by many scientific institutions, especially to determine the mechanism that produces or activates it. But in ancient times, telepathic skills were not interpreted as something normal; they were labeled as devil's talents, black magic, or a demon's activity through a human being, and in some cases they were the cause

---

119   Votre Philodendron est Chatouilleux. Op. cit. pp.70–72.

for people, mostly women, to be considered witches and were burnt alive.

In 1967, the Soviet Maritime News reported, "Cosmonauts when in orbit, seem to be able to communicate telepathically more easily with each other than on Earth. A psychic faculty training system has been incorporated in the cosmonaut training program". During the Apollo 14 mission in 1971 a telepathic experiment (supposedly not authorized by the National Aeronautics and Space Administration NASA), was conducted by Astronaut Edgar D. Mitchell with four recipients on Earth, 150,000 miles below. It proved distance is not a barrier. The experiment was not announced until the mission was completed. In another experiment known as the "Nautilius Affair" the French magazine Constellation published a feature called "Thought Transmission - Weapon of War," which claimed that telepathic experiments were conducted from the US Nautilus (first nuclear submarine) while submerged below the North Pole artic ice (Sunshine mission) transmitting information to people located miles away on shore. That report was followed in February 1960, by a more detailed treatment by Gerald Messadié in "Science et vie,". The US government denied such occurrence (probably by strategic reasons).

Clairvoyance and Retro cognition

The term *clairvoyance* (from French *clair*, meaning "clear" and *voyance*, meaning "vision") is defined as the ability to gain information about an object, person, location, or physical event through means other than the known human normal senses. Because normal senses are not involved in this type of perception, it is included in the group of extrasensory perceptions. So-called *clairvoyants* have been reported in many cultures since ancient times, known for their supernatural ability to perceive events, facts, or objects in a different time (past or future) or beyond normal sensory contact (hidden or distant). Clairvoyance has been historically linked to divination and prophesying. People with such capacities have been known through history with different names, like seers, prophets, forecasters, diviners, soothsayers, clairvoyants, oracles, fortune-tellers, and psychics. Spiritualists call them mediums[120]. The typical image of a clairvoyant is someone sitting in front of a crystal ball.

Unfortunately, as with the other capacities, there are people that pretend to have this capacity (or had it in their past) and use this reputation to promote scams and deceive naive people by charging fees in exchange for supposed information on future events.

To normal clairvoyance could be added *remote viewing*, which is basically a variety of clairvoyance in which an "observer" selects or is given a distant or remote "target" in order to observe it and describe details and activities. This procedure, supposedly, had been used by the US intelligence services as well as the Russian and Chinese espionage. The CIA is said to have conducted a program called *Stargate* that used individuals with remote viewing capacities for intelligence purposes. Today researchers at the Farsight Institute in Atlanta, Georgia, are studying and following past experiences in this field[121].

In order for researchers to explore the nature of the remote-viewing channel, the viewer in some experiments was secured in a double-walled, copper-screened Faraday cage. Although this provided attenuation of radio signals over a broad range of frequencies, the researchers found that it did not alter the subject's remote viewing capability. They postulated that extremely low frequency (ELF) propagation might be involved, since Faraday cage screening is less effective in the ELF range.

The debate about the veracity of clairvoyance, remote viewing, and retro cognition is constant. I understand that many people still have doubts about this phenomenon, but our experience shows that doubting people cease to be so when they have their own experiences that cannot be explained by just alleging randomness and fortuitous coincidences. As I understand, and many people surely share my idea, time is more subjective than objective, and in some way we are supposed to go back and forth at will in that dimension. It is like opening a book

---

120 See *The Book on Mediums* by Alan Kardec.
121 More details on their website: www.farsight.org.

to any page at random and knowing that the pages before it contained past actions in the novel and any page after it will contain its related or following future.

In order for clairvoyance to be possible, and to be able to access past or future information, we need to go outside our time-space frame or dimension, which means going into a dimension where there is no time or space as we know it. From such a position, we could observe events regardless of their time sequencing. Sounds crazy, doesn't it? But pay attention to the following example, which will enable you to better understand the concept. Suppose you are arriving at a train station when a train is departing, and you can observe it from a distance. Its departure speed is slow, which allows you to watch it better. One of the passengers arrived quite late and boarded one of the last coaches just in time. He is moving through the train from the last car to the front one, where his girlfriend, who thinks he missed the train, is sitting. You as a distant observer are located in a different "time-space," where you can observe the passenger in the last wagon and simultaneously his girlfriend in the first. For you, both of them are in your present time. Nevertheless the moving passenger can neither see nor find his girlfriend; he hopes and intends to meet her in his own future time. By the same token, the girl seated in the front coach does not realize that her friend is coming to meet her, a happening that remains possible but not certain in her future time. Both were unaware of their future time when they finally encountered each other. But for you, it is different, as you were watching simultaneously their present times (what is actually happening) *and* their past time (which were the positions they had when the train departed), and you could foresee their future time (because you already knew they would meet in the front coach). That is what it is like to be out of regular time-space and observe events from a different time-space.

A friend of mine clarified the same concept in another simple way. Although it is not the most accurate scientific approach, it is easier to understand. He said to imagine a strip of film, the kind used extensively in cinemas and that is being replaced by digital projectors. If we take the strip between our hands and observe it against a light source, we could watch a scene before, during, and after its occurrence. It could be a cowboy taking his pistol from his holster, shooting, and running away. As an outsider located in another time-space, we are able to see all of this. But the person seated in the movie theater can only follow the sequence and cannot anticipate the future scene.

Tragic events that made big headlines, like the attack on the World Trade Center in 2001, the tsunami in Japan in 2011, or the previous one in Indonesia in 2004[122], revealed that thousands of people had premonitions or visions anticipating those events. The huge quantity of reports indicates that these are not coincidences and were thus the product of a certain type of communication transcending the time and space barriers. There is no way to discard or ignore so many testimonies. To use a quote from Abraham Lincoln, "You can fool all the people some of the time, and some of the people all the time, but you cannot fool all the people all the time."

There is a third type of clairvoyance-related phenomena known as *retro cognition*, by which people know exact details about events in the remote past even though they were not participants or involved in any way. This capacity has been used by many who claim to be psychic investigators and who help police departments solve difficult crimes. This application is also known as *forensic telepathy*.

A famous Dutch psychic named Gerard Croisset helped police solve many cases by applying what some call *psychometrics*. This involves inducing a state in which access to retro cognition occurs by taking in hand an object that was linked to the fact or event. Another notable psychic who helped the police was Pieter van der Hurk (Peter Hurkos), who appears in many documented reports of the police department of Miami, Florida. People with these powers have been reported by hundreds, and many police departments keep records of

---

122   This, also known as Indian Ocean Tsunami, South Asia Tsunami, Indonesian Tsunami, Christmas Tsunami, and Boxing Day Tsunami, on Dec. 26, 2004, caused between approximately 230,000 and 280,000 deaths.

their proceedings. For further reading, I recommend the book *Psychic Detective Stories and Exercises for the Soul*[123].

We've all likely had many experiences in which a *time leap* (or *quantum leap*)[124] was involved. However, we probably did not pay adequate attention when they occurred. Research institutions have been engaged in finding explanations for the causes and origin of those paranormal experiences, and they have gathered in their files thousands of cases in which many events were predicted. Given our deep-rooted concept of a linear time sequence, such abnormal situations disrupt our beliefs and our concept of reality, in which there should be a chronological sequence of before, now, and after.

I could tell you about some of my experiences that could be considered as *leaps into the future* or *progressions*. At the time they occurred, they seemed irrelevant. At most they merely suggested that peering into the future could be possible. Many people do not pay any attention to such events, and most of the time, doing so has no consequences. The only reason I could find to justify those events is that they might be a sort of bizarre distortion in our normal, linear time-space, whose causes or motivations remain unknown to us. I think that these occurrences cannot be considered dèjá vu [[125]] because in fact one *has* already seen the scene, even if it was only in a dream, and it can be clearly remembered. And that is why later on, when one is confronted with real objects and places, they seem to be quite familiar. It may be, however, that when the time lapse between the dream and the real experience is quite long, the person may have almost forgotten the original image and thus think he or she has experienced dèjá vu. I do not know if these unimportant leaps into the future can be classified in the *premonitory* group, for they do

---

123 *Psychic Detective Stories and Exercises for the Soul* by Nancy Orlen Weber (Unlimited Mind Communications Inc., a Division of NOW Inc.).

124 A quantum leap is a leap from A to B without passing through any of the points between A and B. The quantum leap idea works just as well in 2 to 3 dimensions. Something performs a quantum leap if it goes directly from some point A to some other point B without passing through any other points from the time it left A to the time it arrived at B.

125 *Dèjá vu*, from French, literally *"already seen"* is the phenomenon of believing that a present event or experience has occurred in the past.

not present any kind of warning, and it is difficult to assess at the time whether the event is something that could really happen afterward.

In my first experience of this type that I can recall, I had a dream in which I was visiting a medieval castle with a small group of people, and we were going up a hidden spiral staircase. We arrived at a level where we could see old-fashioned marble bathrooms, and there was a balcony opening onto a great hall where there was a wind organ like those that were used in old churches. Surprisingly, a few days later I visited Casa Loma, a big mansion in Toronto, Canada. Though it was built around 1910, it is a replica of a medieval castle.

I had another dream experience, where I was standing in front of a futuristic construction that was unknown to me. I knew that I was in the city of Paris at dusk. The building was made of glass and had white aluminum frames. It was very modern, with many geometric angles and curves. The dream was very real, with a background traffic noise, the chill of a cold wind blowing, and everything in full color and three dimensions. After waking up the next morning and while remembering the dream, I thought it was a fantasy produced by my mind or something of a distant future. This second consideration I discounted because the Paris in the dream was not the city I remembered from real life. But to my surprise that dream became real a few months later when I was visiting Paris again on a business trip after many years of absence. My business partner took me to a well-known *creperie* quite close to the Pompidou Center of Arts, and we had to cross a mall called Forum des Halles, which was built in an area where previously there had been a well-known open market with the same name.

We entered the mall because he wanted to show me where an annex to the Grevin Wax Museum had opened whose original site is in the Grand Boulevards. As I entered the mall, the images I had seen in my dream a few months before were revived in my conscious mind, and I was able to see the astonishing connection between the two. It was a real déjà vu experience that nearly paralyzed me, so much that my friend thought something was wrong with me. I told him politely that I was simply surprised by the beauty of the place without telling him anything else, which would have been awkward for me to do. In fact it is not the same to tell about events than to experience them in our own flesh and bones.

These time leaps or premonitions could be perceived long before an event or at short notice. I clearly remember one of latter. I was in Cincinnati, Ohio, on a business trip, and our supplier made a reservation for me in a motel not far from their factory. I arrived late in the afternoon and was supposed to meet my counterpart the next day for breakfast and a factory visit. That night I had an unusual dream in which I was walking around a pool where there was a Mexican hat made out of stone or concrete and painted with colors. The day after, upon remembering the dream, I laughed because of the absurdity of the object, but in a dream anything is possible. To my surprise the next day I had to cross a yard to get to the restaurant, and there was a pool, which could not be seen from my room on the opposite side. Of course, this was something to be expected in such a motel, but the very same weird stone Mexican hat I'd saw in my dream the night before was there, too. For me that was an unexpected surprise and also a kind of irrelevant time leap. Though the dream of the hat and the actual sighting of it occurred within just a few hours of each other, it was indeed a time leap, or what others refer to as a quantum leap. Events like these have helped many people to avoid accidents and save their own and others' lives. I think that most of us have had plenty of similar experiences, but due to their seeming irrelevance, they have been forgotten. These experiences are similar to those times I've encountered a friend on the street who assures me that, although it is difficult to believe, he had just been thinking about me. Or when we call someone out of the blue and the person on the other end remarks that he was just thinking about us when the phone rang. All these types of experiences are indeed spontaneous, but with due practice and guidance, these experiences could be produced at will.

The combination of Qigong procedures with our available innate mental powers (or potential capacity) allow us to cross the barrier of time in either direction, to the past or the future.

Thousands of years ago in India, the *Yoga Sutras* of Patanjali exposed a teaching that had without any doubt a component of modern quantum physics regarding our time-space dimension:

> ## Kaivalya Pada IV-12
> ### Atîtặnặgatam svarûpato 'sty ashva-bhedặd
> "The past and future exist in their own way (real). Different properties (*dharma*) depend on the difference of the way."

This in essence means that time is subjective and that our feelings change its perception. The ancient religious scriptures such as the Christian Bible and Jewish Torah, as well as different texts in Islam and Buddhism, are full of historical documentation of events attributed to prophets who could anticipate and see future events (i.e. cross the time barrier). Today many people do the same outside any religious environment. I would call this shared experience as "planetary" for having appeared in different cultures around the world and at different times.

In the process of regression under hypnosis, which basically is an induced altered state of consciousness, we travel in time to the past. But other feelings traveling to the past or future may occur outside the framework of hypnosis. These are spontaneous (as opposed to induced), either in a vision, a dream, or in a real-time perception, as when we see some place, person, or object that seems already known to us.

Research institutions' files and data compilation are full of stories that involve a documented mental transfer forward to the future or backward to the past. With such evidence scientists are presented with the task of determining the mechanism that allows humans to perceive events that transcend time barriers. But they are also facing a situation that poses some difficult questions: If we can perceive the future and then we can verify that our perception was real, then is everything already determined? Is there a fate that cannot be changed?

The answer could be found in the so-called quantum theory, which tells us that all events are not linked to a simple linear sequence that ends in a final, predetermined outcome. Instead, at the end multiple possibilities coexist, and it is only the action of our free will that can lead us to one of them through different ways. This theory explains why a premonition can still be considered a premonition even if the event never occurs. For instance, one may have a premonition of an accident and then, because of the premonition, change the plans and so avoid the accident. How could the person perceive the event and then avoid the accident if the person was not really present in that location at the time as perceived in the premonitory vision? Qigong, raja-yoga, and other procedures that are carried out during an altered state of consciousness allow us a glimpse of the past and the future. People who perceive these extraordinary events have no doubt that they are in fact realities in other time frames, but they cannot explain why this is possible. It is something beyond their knowledge, and to most people it remains a mystery.

In relation to clairvoyance and the influence this has had on the discovery of ruins and lost civilizations, a new branch of science has been created that has been called *psychic archeology* (or intuitive archeology), which attempts to locate missing or buried underground places, constructions, or artifacts, through a mental leap in time (retro cognition). Many documented accounts exist of archaeological findings where intuition or retro cognition have provided a valuable contribution to the discoveries. For example, Mr. George Mc Mullen, an intuitive archeologist has assisted many archeologists around the world, giving correct information about prehistoric Canada, ancient Egypt, and the Middle East, details that were confirmed by subsequent research and findings. Another intuitive archeologist was Stefan Ossowiecki[126], and other professional archeologists who introduced psychic searching methods are, among others, Frederick Bligh Bond, Tom Lethbridge, and J. Norman Emerson[127] (1917–1978).

Sometimes I wonder how our relationship with time works. Is it like a computer game, where multiple possibilities are already there waiting for our decisions? Which one of these possibilities will materialize, and how? Do our present actions change future results? Or rather are we subject to what is known as the fate or something that "was written."

Clairaudience

Clairaudience is the sonic equivalent of clairvoyance. Some people report that they have heard voices in particular circumstances. They report having received messages of unknown origin from persons associated with them, either alive or dead. I've had this experience, too, although sporadically. These messages received in the form of voices have intrigued me, and at times I have questioned myself by considering these events symptoms of a mental illness. But I recently saw a documentary in which people with schizophrenia claimed to hear voices. It was initiated a neurological study, and it could establish that these people actually were receiving a signal in the brain that would be the equivalent of a voice, but not from the sound receptors (the ears). Instead the source of the voices was the human language center (in the brain). That is, it was found out what was obvious: a part of the brain is used as a transducer to change neurotransmitters' pulse signals into a verbal code of words. It was clear that the voices did not come from outside, as any sound that is like a vibration of air. But the documentary did not reveal where the nerve stimulus acting on the language centers of the brain came from.

---

126 See *A World in a Grain of Sand: The Clairvoyance of Stefan Ossowieski* by Ian Stevenson, Zofia Weaver, and Mary Rose Barrington.

127 J. Norman Emerson was a Canadian archaeologist based out of Toronto with a doctorate from Chicago. He was one of the big names in North American archaeology and President of the Canadian Archaeological Association, 1970.

So, in short, to hear voices is not a symptom of madness based on the fact that these do not occur from a physical, material sound outside our body. They are a form of perception through "other channels" that stimulate the language centers of the brain, located in the frontal lobe (which explains why they are considered extrasensory perception). One must consider the difference between mentally generated voices and physically generated voices. To produce the latter requires enough energy for the air to vibrate with such intensity that we may hear it. In addition the air would have to vibrate at very specific frequencies to replicate a voiceprint of someone in particular, since it has been determined that each voice is unique, leaving a print similar to a fingerprint (which is why voiceprints are used to track police callers or to identify people in recorded communications).

It actually requires less effort and energy to generate and perceive a weak signal that the brain transforms into words and that has the characteristics of those who sent or transmitted them (i.e. to carry the voiceprint). Consider a radio signal that carries the voice of our favorite singer or a television signal carrying the colors of the costumes. It is well documented and proven that our brain has the ability to receive telepathic transmissions, so it is not that strange that it may receive a signal that is processed in the language centers of the brain as familiar voices. The real problem is to determine where the signal comes from, and in which way.

OBEs, Astral Projection, and Bilocation

On the scale of development and progress, the next step is extracorporeal experiences, or OBEs (out-of-body experiences), which are of two types. The first is an individual event, virtual, that takes place in the mind or thoughts of the person. The subject feels as if he or she is moving out of his or her physical body to other places, voluntarily or spontaneously. This is also known as *astral travel* or *astral projection*. In the second type, a physical bodily relocation occurs. This is no longer an individual feeling or experience but is shared by external witnesses.

Let's look at the following example. If two witnesses standing at different points identify a criminal, those reports have a great value for police investigators as evidence. In fact, the more witnesses, the greater the proofing value because all witnesses in different locations could not be all mistaken at the same time, so any matches or coinciding reports are considered as evidence. I mention this because I am very skeptical about third-party retellings, and I do not take plainly the stories I've found in Qigong books about people being present in two places at the same time. But if these events are reported by several people located in different places and under different circumstances, those versions reinforce one another, giving credence to the original story. Remarkably, not only Chinese reported these phenomena, but Christian religious texts report many examples of this type of experience, called *bilocation* and generally attributed to saints.

For Catholics, bilocation is the simultaneous presence of the same person in two different places. There have been numerous cases of such in the lives of the saints. The most notable are Pope Saint Clement, Saint Francis of Assisi, Saint Anthony of Padua, Saint Francis Javier, Saint Martin of Porres, Saint Joseph of Cupertino, Saint Alphonsus Liguori, Saint John Bosco, and, recently, the Blessed Father Pio of Pietrelcina. Outside the context of Qigong similar cases have also been reported, like that of the Buddhist monk Milarepa.

I had the opportunity to read a translated report in which a Qigong master told a group of present witnesses that he would teletransport himself to a train station located about eighty miles away and requested that the station chief be called to verify that he had indeed moved to that place. He disappeared out of sight, and the witnesses called the station chief, as requested. The master was really there, and the chief put him on the phone. The remarkable thing is that the master, having demonstrated his unusual capability, then returned by train, a detail that, by the way, provided additional proof of his presence in the distant place. I think that his return by normal means was partly due to the fact that these phenomena consume a lot of energy; there might not have been enough remaining energy for him to return the same way. It would be like traveling in a car to a remote place where it was not possible to refill the gas tank and having to return by other means.

Catholics agree with the Taoists that bilocation can be of two different types, the first purely in spirit (which would be as a projection) and the second in body and soul, or matter and energy (i.e., the whole person). The Taoists describe this latter phenomena resulting either from the *ying-shen* or from *yang-shen*, in which *shen* is the word to describe the spirit. So it could be a positive bilocation (ying-sheng) or a full relocation (yang-shen). In both cases the teletransported entity has all the characteristics of the original physical body in shape, volume, appearance, and vitality. In other cases, the transfer is not complete, and the image seen is a transparent, ghostly type projected image.

According to Catholics, when bilocation is performed only in spirit and is observed just as a projection or appearance (without physical matter), the physical presence of the person remains, or continues, in the starting point, and in the site where the projection takes place, the image is purely representative (visible as a body). Otherwise when bilocation is done in body and soul (matter and energy)[128], the presence of the person is physical where the body is observed as a visible presence, while at the site that the person leaves, what remains is a pictorial form (a projection). This dual presence, representative on one side and physical on the other, is essential to the bilocation phenomena in whatever way it occurs. A person has never been reported to have been in both places in body and soul (matter and energy) at the same time: this is impossible. However, witnesses could be mistaken by the projection seen in one of the locations. It should also be stressed that this double presence, in order to be considered a true bilocation requires transportation (i.e., the moving of a person from one place to another) either in body and soul or in spirit. In both alternatives, the ability to interact simultaneously in the two separate environments is also required.

---

128 Because the third component, the spirit, is nonlocal and not time bound

Psychokinesis and Structural Changes in Matter

Another development achieved by the practice of Qigong is the increased psychokinetic[129] power, which is the outcome observed on physical objects (moving, breaking, and so on) triggered by enhanced mental intent during an altered state. Such events in extreme cases might produce materialization, disappearance, or even structural changes. But in any case this activity involves the action of unknown forces that make the objects in question either move or be changed. Like the other capacities, Psychokinesis is highly debatable. In addition, it has been exploited endlessly in science fiction movies and TV series dealing with themes of magic, spells, and fairy tales, which is a contributing reason for the disbelief of many people.

Skeptics have often stated that moving objects in the air or human levitation is impossible because it is contrary to the law of universal gravitation. They say that those who have witnessed some kind of levitation might have been under a kind of mental illusion. Scientific advances take time, but they do develop and slowly surpass perplexing thresholds. A frog levitating in the air? Reality or illusion? Well, this was a reality in an experiment developed by researchers in the super magnet at the National High Magnetic Field Laboratory (NHMFL) at Florida State University in Tallahassee. They also submitted plants of the genus Arabidopsis to magnetic levitating periods to study the effects on genes. Although about 9.4 Tesla was necessary to make the frog levitate in the laboratory of the NHMFL,[130] that magnetic field is stronger than the earth's magnetic field (1 Tesla is about 20,000 times stronger). There are other conditions for structural changes of matter that could achieve the same effect with lower magnetic fields and with the support of other forces.

---

129 Psychokinesis (from Greek ψυχή κίνησις, translated as "mind movement") or telekinesis (Greek τ☐λε κίνησις, "distant movement") is an alleged psychic ability allowing a person to influence an external physical system without physical interaction. Psychokinesis and telekinesis are sometimes abbreviated as PK and TK, respectively

130 See the web page of the NHMFL: www.magnet.fsu.edu.

Advances in technology have brought Psychokinesis to the forefront of laboratory tests. The extraordinary Russian psychics Nelya Kulagina and Alla Vinogradova[131] conducted countless experiments in which they were able to move small objects without physical contact. One of the most striking laboratory experiments related to the control of matter and energy by commands of the control element (the mind, or spirit) was performed by Kulagina and led by the neuro physicist Genady Sergeyev in the Utomskii Institute in Leningrad[132]. Sergeyev broke the shell of an egg and poured its contents into an aquarium filled with a saline solution and instructed Kulagina to separate the yolk from the white. Over a period of thirty minutes, slowly Kulagina was able to separate the egg apart at a distance and then agglutinate the yolk. The lab reports that this effort left Kulagina exhausted and almost blind. Her pulse rose to 240 beats per minute, and her blood sugar level rose significantly, as such level tends to do in any stressful situation. Reported as well was the loss of nearly one kilo of weight, which indicated a strong energy transfer.

Under normal conditions, people are able to change the structure and properties of some elements by introducing variations in temperature, time, pressure, or tension. Metals, for example, are melted and molded at high temperatures, and if pressure is applied, they can also be deformed. Some chemical reactions achieved by adding compounds of a different type or radiation can change matter properties as well. Recent research allows us to state that the application of qi by the method of Qigong is also able to alter the structural properties of some materials.

Experiments conducted by Dr. Yan and colleagues in May 1998 at the Research Institute of Hydro-Physics in Beijing, China, in cooperation with the Qigong master Mr. Ou Wen Wai, demonstrated that qi is a form of energy that produces significant structural changes in water and aqueous substances, alters the phase behavior of liposomes DPPC[133], and allows growth of crystals of Fab protein.

---

131 *Super-Minds* by John Taylor. New York: Viking Press, 1975 (pp. 38, 39).
132 *Secrets of the Inner Mind.* Time-Life Books, Alexandria, Virginia,– 1993.
133 (Dipalmitoyl-phosphatidyl-choline)

In a course of Qigong that I conducted several years ago, we conducted some experiments on matter's property changes. The first was done with a couple of bottles of Manischewitz (Kosher) wine, which is produced in the United States. We took one bottle to apply Qigong and set the other apart as a control sample. Both bottles were opened and offered to those present for wine tasting, and all agreed that there was no difference in taste between the two. At the conclusion of the period of qi application, we proceeded to taste both the "treated" wine and the control sample. The participants noticed a considerable difference in the degree of sweetness (Manischewitz is a sweet wine made out of concord grapes), and it was noticed as well that the treated wine had a floral aroma that previously was absent. All agreed and choose as the better wine that which had undergone treatment, and some even commented that possibly it would have acquired special properties. The matter of treating an object with the power of intention is not mere superstition, though many people use the term *energy* carelessly, ignoring the principles that govern it. In laboratory experiments the capacity to alter the molecular structure (not atomic) of many materials is well proven.

The Christian Bible narrates an interesting episode of structural transformation of matter. In the Gospel according to Saint John[134], he narrates an episode during a wedding in Canaan, where Jesus' mother said to him that there was no more wine. Then Jesus said to the servants to fill the jars with water, and it was transformed into wine. It is reported that the master of the banquet tasted the water that had been turned into wine, not knowing where it had come from, and he told the bridegroom that everyone usually brings out the choice wine first and then the cheaper wine after the guests have had too much to drink.

Many so-called miracles performed by Jesus of Nazareth have been considered by his opponents to be fables or fancies of his followers. But Qigong and its associated experiments clearly show that such miracles could be performed by a powerful spirit. A normal human, with proper

---

134 St. John 2, 1,11

training, can make small but significant changes, and this provides an indication of what can be achieved by more advanced and powerful spirits.

Qigong masters (Shifu) like Ou Wen Wai have also changed the properties of red wine. Before issuing qi the absorption peak was 278.4 nanometers (nm) and 1277 A (Absorbance index). Then after issuing qi the absorption peak of the treated wine was 278.4 nm and 1.230 A. The difference of 0.047 A showed a change in the concentration. This experience of Master Ou Wen, reinforces our humble experience when changing the properties of that Manischewitz wine. I also have a video in which the Master Chen Lin Fen from the Wisdomics Association of Beijing changes the acidity level (pH) of a liquid substance. In the experiment a digital measuring instrument (pH meter)[135] was immersed in the liquid, and the figures on the screen began to vary, indicating that the liquid was yielding to a significant change in pH. Also in the same video is an experiment that changes the standard frequency of a frequency generator instrument with ruby crystal. These devices are so precise that they are used as standards to calibrate other less precise devices; nevertheless, Master Chen managed to change some few thousandths of the precise pattern generated by the ruby crystal.

During that same Qigong course, on another occasion, I asked participants each to bring to class a 500 ml (aprox. 16 oz.) bottle of physiological saline solution (the type used in hospitals), which were then submitted to treatment (or "charging") with Qigong. I told the participants that they could use the treated solution for cosmetic purposes, such as washing the face with the serum and cleaning areas of skin that had problems such as roughness or fungal stains. The men were advised to use it as aftershave. A couple of weeks later, participants were asked to narrate their experiences with the treated saline solution, and all reported results were highly positive. In some cases the solution had cured small, superficial skin lesions. The men said it was the best

---

135 A pH meter is an electronic device used for measuring the pH (acidity or alkalinity) of a liquid (though special probes are sometimes used to measure the pH of semisolid substances).

aftershave they had used: it cooled their faces, seemed to heal small cuts, and produced skin rejuvenation. After this experience the participants asked me to repeat the experiment to replenish their depleted supply, but we did not, for the intention of the experiment was only to observe the change that occurred in the matter. Our experience with saline solution is reinforced by reports on an experience of Master Ou. He also found obvious differences in salt solutions—precisely measured with an infrared spectrograph—before and after the issuance of qi.

Minor alterations induced by the emission of qi are also able to prevent the aging, corrosion, and deterioration caused by weather and external agents on metals, preventing their oxidation. I myself usually use disposable shavers (the cheapest), but to the dismay of manufacturers, these often last me for several months without damage. I even had one that lasted almost nine months, and the cause it did not last longer was that I lost it on a trip. For the peace of the manufacturers, I can assure them that I have not released the treatment method I use, so their sales will not be substantially diminished.

During the altered mental states used to enhance the intentionality of actions on material objects by manipulating energy, as used in Qigong, people reported variations and patterns that have been subjected to intense laboratory verification processes with surprising results. Often these phenomena are attributed to superminds or super endowed people, but this is not entirely accurate. Each person is able to operate such phenomena through proper training, and proof of this is the existence of methods such as Qigong. Had Qigong not produced results, over time people would have forgotten the procedure. What happens with these energy-control methods is that some people have more innate ability than others, as is the case for athletes, musicians, writers, and the like. Just as a music school will produce normal musicians and great songwriters or interpreters, likewise with Qigong training some will become masters and others simple performers.

Qigong texts are not the only where the ability to alter the properties and structure of matter has been reliably documented. The Yogis of India and the so-called psychics of today have also reported such events. Among multiple effects, one has been named: the Geller effect[136] that occurs when people bend, twist, and break metal spoons and forks. Physicist John Taylor, who specialized in particle physics, cosmology, and brain research, published an excellent work called *Super Minds*[137], the content of which undermines traditional principles of physics in terms of changing the properties of matter.

In research conducted on metal pieces already bent by Uri Geller, these were submitted to metallographic and spectroscopic study. Although structural changes could be observed in the crystals, their joints had not been altered, as would occur in a process using high temperatures. More out of curiosity than anything else, I did an experiment with some friends by attempting to bend a steel fork with the action of Qigong (without applying physical force). To my surprise, the steel bent before our eyes. Since then I've kept that fork in my desk drawer as a conversation piece on the subject. I am not a supporter of the shows in which some individuals attempt to demonstrate to others certain supposedly extraordinary abilities to arouse admiration and awe. As I have already stated, these abilities are not unique: they belong to all humans who, through proper training, could make use of them with varying degrees of results.

---

136 From the name of the Israeli psychic Uri Geller.
137 Taylor, John. *Super-Minds*. New York: Viking Press, 1975.

At Princeton University in New Jersey, a program known as Princeton Engineering Anomalies Research (PEAR)[138] was established in 1979 by Robert G. Jahn, who at the time was Dean of the faculty of engineering and applied sciences. This program was developed to scientifically and rigorously study the interaction and influence of the human mind or psyche on sensitive physical devices and systems or procedures currently applied in normal engineering processes.

There is another phenomenon that I do not know how to classify: invisibility. In real life this phenomenon does not occur in the fantastic way shown in the movies. It is rather a simple blocking of the visual field or perception of the observer (i.e., the person becomes invisible only to the targeted observer but remains visible to others, since the body is still physically present). After some time of invisibility, the surrounding persons or animals can perceive again the image. Often they could be quite surprised or scared because they do not know where the previous invisible person came from. "Being invisible" is not to be confused with physical disappearance. On many occasions I have experienced this process for a very short time with people and animals, and because we do not really disappear the effects could only be detected by the reactions of the surrounding person or animal.

Many times these extraordinary or paranormal phenomena are not the intended outcome of the practice of Qigong. Often they are but a by-product or collateral effect from the increased powers obtained in the practice. This is due to the qi energy being manipulated by our control element (spirit). People who begin to practice Qigong usually don't do it for the purpose of becoming magicians; in fact, there comes a time when

---

138 The Princeton Engineering Anomalies Research (PEAR) program, which flourished for nearly three decades under the aegis of Princeton University's School of Engineering and Applied Science, has completed its experimental agenda of studying the interaction of human consciousness with sensitive physical devices, systems, and processes, and developing complementary theoretical models to enable better understanding of the role of consciousness in the establishment of physical reality. PEAR has now incorporated its present and future operations into the broader venue of the ICRL, a 501(c)(3) not-for-profit research organization, in addition to Psyleron—a company that provides Random Event Generator devices to enable the continued exploration of PEAR's findings by the general public and research communities

all the phenomenal aspects begin to fade into the background. They are considered normal, not given any importance, not worth to constantly repeat them, and even avoided in some cases.

The Taoists explain that one who is dedicated to the cultivation and development of paranormal powers before achieving wisdom can easily be diverted, and they call this the "black" way, or the way of wrong thoughts. Such individuals will lose not only their powers but their original objectives as well. Further, Taoists say that those who use their powers to entertain or fascinate others follow the path of *mara*, the way that impedes self-progress and the progress of others, also defined as an incorrect point of view resulting from external psychological or physiological influences.

We could compare this situation to that already mentioned of bodybuilders who, worried about their health and physical bodies, become slaves to an idea. They dedicate all their time to improving the body's shape and outer appearance, overshadowing the original purpose of achieving a balanced and healthy life.

CHAPTER 18

Qigong and Spirituality

For many readers this chapter will be somewhat controversial and difficult to grasp because it goes against certain established principles that have become dogmas in different organized religions, almost none of which accept that anyone could challenge the rules imposed on its followers.

The purpose of this book is not to discuss religious issues that are controversial and a source of constant conflict. I just want to make clear that many of the effects that have been observed since the time of witches and shamans (the same that religions have used to attract followers) are in fact the result of a capacity inherent to human nature. Organized religions, which I think all of them are to a greater or lesser degree, often impose on their followers a set of rules they must observe or otherwise risk penalties in this life or, even worse, in the afterlife. It is a form of control in the name of God.

The basis of the teachings in the Jewish religion is the Torah, which is equivalent to the Christian Bible In fact both share many books of the Old Testament. But the rabbis have added the Talmud, a collection of laws, regulations, or binding orders. For Islam, the irrefutable source is the Holy Koran (Al Qur'an Al Karim), but the religion also has imposed a number of mandatory requirements known as *Sharia*[139] (or Shariah), the Islamic law that dictates misdemeanors, offenses, and punishments.

In the remote past, when much of the world's population was completely illiterate and ignorant and had no access to written documents, it was very easy to be manipulated. Christianity has existed for over two thousand years, but only in recent centuries could Christians read and know a book called the Bible. For fifteen hundred years or more, many generations of Christians were born, grew, and died without ever having access to their main religious text, which besides, was written in a dead foreign language.

I was born and raised in a Catholic family and studied in a Catholic school for nine years. I acknowledge that the moral principles and discipline imposed on us at that time made me a person who cares a great deal about fellow human beings. But I eventually became aware of a number of inconsistencies and absurdities based on blind faith that had been imposed on us. My contacts with other countries, cultures, and religions (due to my work activities) allowed me to compare concepts, mostly accept the ones that coincided with my own knowledge and beliefs, and reject the conflicting ones. I have good friends who belong to different faiths, and we coincide on a lot of topics. But religions have tried to explain some extraordinary phenomena based on obscure knowledge and are fanatically opposed to that which could challenge their inherited teachings and power, even though the origin of such is not 100 percent clear or authenticated. These unfounded explanations have been so diverse that humanity is divided, and the separation has strong cultural and regional roots. All followers are taught that "their religion" is the perfect way to live here and beyond.

Historical chronicles are full of battles between religious groups determined to impose their own version of the truth. Unfortunately in the twenty-first century there is still heavy fighting, not only between

---

139 Shariah is the Islamic canonical law based on the teachings of the Koran and the traditions of the Prophet (Hadith and Sunna), prescribing both religious and secular duties and sometimes retributive penalties for law breaking. The manner in which it should be applied in modern states is a subject of dispute between Islamic fundamentalists and modernists.

groups with completely different beliefs, but also within the same religious or cultural groups, like Sunni and Shiite Muslims or Catholics and Protestants in Ireland and Northern Ireland.

The Christian movement initiated by Jesus of Nazareth and his apostles has been divided into so many denominations that it is hard to count them. There are about twenty-two different denominations that are known as Catholic churches. In total more than 250 denominations are considered non-Catholic Christians, many of which in turn are split into other multiple churches or church confederations based on regional differences or location, and new branches are emerging still. The primary reason there are so many Christian denominations, faiths, or churches is that a lot of their leaders, not agreeing with certain teachings or dogmas, try to impose their own judgment or personal interpretation and end up creating separate groups. In all of those leaders manifests an exaggerated arrogance that makes them take a proudly uncompromising position. In other words, only they are right, and everyone else is wrong. Eastern religions have not escaped these processes, and therefore we can see several different schools of Buddhism and Hinduism.

If God could laugh, as humans do, he would not stop laughing while observing the number of intermediaries who charge ordinary citizens (or request a "contribution") for their services in order these can communicate with him. It's almost like the fee collected by telephone companies. Fortunately God does not have any human qualities, and therefore is not vindictive or spiteful, because if God were so, would have already made them to be disappeared. The warning inherent in the story of Sodom and Gomorrah, cities mentioned in the Bible that were razed by the Lord, is nothing more than a human interpretation that attributes a natural tragedy, perhaps volcanic, to a vengeful being who was said to have punished the people. The ancient Mexican Aztecs and their predecessors the Olmec and Toltec, like the Incas in Peru, interpreted natural phenomena such as droughts or floods as punishment from their gods, and they did not think anything more fitting than to perform human sacrifices to appease these gods. How could a creator be appeased with the destruction of the beings he or she created?

There are many false prophets, self-erected authorized intermediaries of God. And how do we prove their pretense? Supposedly they had a private conversation with the creator. They supposedly were following instructions to create a church with a beautiful name. After that, their fantasy is fulfilled, and so begins the business of living off of others without working.

When I, while studying and practicing Qigong, discovered that many reported miraculous acts were not exclusive to a particular religion or sect and that these acts had been used to manipulate our fellow beings, I became convinced that organized and hierarchical religions are the worst thing that could have happened to humanity. Ignorance favors creation of many sects or cults while illustration opposes them. There are undoubtedly many individuals who make extraordinary social and human contributions and are also members of a religious organization. But their contributions are not by any means the result of their membership in the organization. Rather, it is the conviction, ethics, and dedication of the individual that is responsible for his action. Perhaps the organization, sect, or religion to which a virtuous person belongs may offer him some values that serve as a framework, but, paradoxically, not all members of that faith respect and share those values. Generally speaking, religious organizations appropriate the merit of good deeds done by any of their members and attempt to make them look like a result of their doctrines or principles. It is simple propaganda.

We also see that people who are members of nongovernmental (and nonreligious) organizations make similar social contributions and give great help to their peers. So, clearly, being a member of a religious organization is not a prerequisite for acting in favor of other people in need. The difference between social actions accomplished by religious organizations and social actions accomplished by secular organizations is that secular organizations perform such in solidarity with other members of the human race. Religious organizations, on the other hand, are based on a kind of two-part blackmailing scheme: the first part encourages members by stating that performing such actions makes people earn points to enter a supposed paradise; the second part, which mainly benefits the church, is that such good deeds help spread the faith or belief of the involved religious group.

In general, remember that any organization is a human construction, and systems such as these have as their first priority the survival of the same (i.e., to maintain their existence). This quest for survival is reflected in the actions of their leaders. The collective is important in terms of solidarity, but the group is also a source of power. Just look at the medieval Catholic Church, which appointed and removed the kings in Europe.

To occupy a privileged position in any religious organization requires a collective that supports both the organization and its leaders. God, Allah, Jehovah, Yahweh, Brahma, or whatever name people use, is by definition an omnipotent being, one that does not require intermediaries or guides, especially if these intermediaries are tariffed. Our history is full of examples of bad or evil things done in the name of or in behalf of either the people or God.

One of the problems that we have as thinking beings is that we create mental images or concepts based on what is already known to us. While these can be useful, they become a problem when we try to apply them to planes or dimensions different from ours, where our experiences and realities cannot be transferred. That is likely why humans envision God as someone like themselves, but bigger and more powerful. We, Catholics, have made a great mistake by worshipping the image of a crucified Jesus of Nazareth, which is basically a human body, for we are unwittingly worshiping a human figure. During several centuries, when Christianity first began, followers paid more attention to the teachings than to the human figure of Jesus; at that time the symbol of Christians was a fish

(*Ichthys*)[140], which, by the way, was not the object of adoration or veneration.

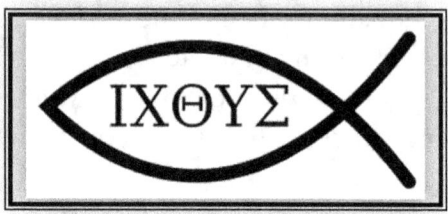

Admittedly a virtue of Islam and of many Evangelic Christian denominations is that they avoid the graphical representation of God and thus unconsciously practicing idolatry (worship and veneration of images of saints and virgins). Anyone who thinks that worshipping images of virgins is not idolatry need only to count the many different virgins that exist in the Catholic world. Each different version (names, clothing, skin color, and so on) is considered the patron of a certain community or region, and she is the only they pay tribute to, ask for miracles, and venerate. The other hundreds of virgins are alien beings who belong to others. And many of those worshipers forget their God in their worship of their virgins.

Qigong is not atheist or agnostic in itself. On the contrary, it allows practitioners to perceive and realize the existence of something higher, something we cannot understand because it's above our level of comprehension. But raising our consciousness to higher levels often makes us rebel against false values instilled by organized religions. When we realize that we can achieve a kind of communion with the entity some call God without the use of intermediaries, we begin to wonder, why do we need them? Why pay them? What is the correct ritual to approach God? What is the correct posture to communicate with God? Should we kneel? Should we face Mecca, the Vatican, the Kremlin, or the White House?

Higher levels in altered states of consciousness reached during practices of Qigong seem not to be the limit or top of mental activity, as there are indications that there is something else beyond. Imagine getting

---

[140] Among the symbols employed by the early Christians, the fish seems to have ranked first in importance. Its popularity among Christians was due principally to the famous acrostic consisting of the initial letters of five Greek words forming the word for fish (*ichthus*), that briefly but clearly described the character of Christ and the claim to worship of believers.

to a high floor in a building, thinking it is the last one, only to realize that there are still other upper levels. However, the elevator doesn't go any higher. In order to go higher, we should take another elevator, one that begins its journey from that level.

Altered states beyond what seems to be the highest level have been described in Qigong and raja-yoga. The number of people who practice Qigong able to reach those levels is extremely low, perhaps one in several thousand. In some practices I've had a chance to peek through a crack and glimpse the entry threshold to that state, and what surprises me is that at the previous level, as a gateway, everything was already extremely clear. All explanations were given; all knowledge was available. There are no mysteries or secrets, just omniscience. Undoubtedly one must fulfill many requirements in order to reach that state. One such requirement is total detachment from people and material possessions, like not belonging to this world despite having a human body. Those who have not yet been able to reach those levels, myself included, can just peek there for a few seconds (seconds that, by the way, seem very long). When we return to our time and dimension, we cannot bring anything with us; all that information with characteristics of omniscience remains on the other side. It's like looking at what the ancients called *akasha*. It's like the memory of having tasted a rich cake that disappears afterwards.

After practicing Qigong for a couple of years or more, which involves access repetitively and constant to altered states of consciousness, the awakening of certain skills that we had previously agreed to call paranormal or, more appropriately, exceptional human abilities occurs. During those states, a phenomenon that some call transcendence is produced. This effect of transcending our reality by contacting our control element (spirit) gives us access to a different dimension; many describe it as spiritual, but it has countless other names according to the cultures or conveniences. It is this type of repeated experience that is known to be a constituent of higher or spiritual Qigong. These experiences are not for everyone, but it is worth knowing about.

Scientists, especially those studying the psyche, are very cautious with the use of the word *spiritual*. They do not like it because they perceive a religious connotation, but they nevertheless recognize that a dimension exists where the subjective and the objective have no boundaries and that scientists have no means to interact experimentally there. We will talk of spirituality related to Qigong as that which is beyond the merely material, cannot be perceived with our normal organs of perception, and is also extremely difficult to describe in words. Whether one refers to the spirit as a higher self, etheric body, supreme mind, higher consciousness, or something else, it does not alter the effects that could be observed. I insist that it is like talking about sun rising: regardless of which language we use to refer to the event, both the light and the heat it provides us are always the same.

Qigong during its development, as we have narrated before, was quite attached to the temples, monasteries, or lamaseries where monks who made a life there belonged to the predominant religious currents (i.e., Taoist or Buddhist). We can say in general terms that the monks when entering convents were in search of spiritual and not material outcomes. Many of them did not seek economic survival or practical living solutions; their intention was to have access to a group or sect that could assure them a kind of permanent higher state known as enlightenment. These supreme enlightenment states were known in Zen Buddhism as *satori* or *kenshou*, in Theravada Buddhism as *arhat*, in Mahayana Buddhism as *bodhisattva*, in Tibetan Buddhism as *dzogchen*, in Hinduism as *moksha* or *nirvana*, and in Taoism as a kind of immortality.

In Western culture and Abrahamic monotheistic religions, there is no precise equivalent. For example, in the Catholic religion, people speak of a state of holiness, but usually this refers to a postmortem situation. The Sufis, an esoteric branch of Islam, accept reaching a similar state that is considered a continuous divine remembrance or *dhikr*.

Many have tried in vain to put into words the characteristics of enlightenment, and I think there is much confusion about it, especially because it is a subjective experience. My skeptical side has noticed that many strange things happened in those temples, some of them true, some legends, and some terrible misunderstandings. So not all that could be described as enlightenment was really such a thing. In this analysis we have to consider that medical knowledge in ancient times were very rudimentary, and sometimes it happened that a person fell into a physical and mental disorder due to many circumstances that concurred to show an abnormal behavior, but such conduct was prone to any interpretation.

Some monks could have undergone strict diets for long periods of time that put their bodies out of chemical balance, perhaps for lack or deficiency of electrolytes such as sodium, potassium, and magnesium. Other monks could have had problems with strokes and as result remained practically catatonic, and their colleagues may have thought this was a sign of having achieved enlightenment or supreme consciousness.

When a monk would tarry for several days, sitting in front of a wall without speaking or moving, it was considered a great achievement. Instead of providing medical assistance, the monks would celebrate. There is no doubt that due to their ignorance they engaged in processes of intensive fasting beyond the limits the human body can endure. These undermined their health and induced all kinds of hallucinations, which were erroneously interpreted as visions from the afterlife. I do not think it's a simple coincidence that most of the alleged divine revelations reported by many mystics in different religions, including Christians, have occurred after long fasting periods.

Other times, when any of the older monks spoke incoherently and incomprehensibly, such conduct was interpreted as the expressions of a great wisdom that novices or disciples were not yet able to clearly understand. Today a person in similar circumstances would be taken to a hospital with signs of stroke. Many monks associated the term *enlightenment* with the perception of intense white light whose source could not be explained. But quite possibly they were suffering from hypoxia, or significant lack of oxygen, which causes feeling of being in the presence of an intense white lights at the end of a tunnel (similar to experiences people recount after having undergone cardiac resuscitation, falsely interpreted as being dead and returning to life). It is the same effect as the one perceived by military test pilots when exposed to intense forces of centrifugal acceleration in flight simulators or when performing actual maneuvers at high altitudes. But pilots do not say they reached a state of enlightenment.

This is something to keep in mind so as to not believe all the things that are attributed to certain persons by alleged eyewitnesses who have only heard the subjective explanation and were unable to understand the objective and physiological part due to lack of knowledge. Unfortunately over time some fantastic tales have endured attributed to supposed protagonists in ancient China, stories that were further distorted in the chain of oral transmission through many people over an extremely long period.

Buddhism is deeply rooted in China, where it shares its preeminence with Taoism and Confucianism. In most temples and monasteries of those faiths Qigong was a common practice, and we can observe that many of its teachings are similar to those coming from India. That is why the higher Qigong, the one in search of enlightenment, coincides in its methods with Buddhism, and Zen Buddhism (Charn) and somehow also with Hinduism, to which they are all related. This connection has been lost in time, and it is very difficult to determine in what proportion the different philosophical groups are influenced by one another. Only the passage of time and further research may determine the original influence of Buddhism on Qigong.

Thanks to a friend of the higher Lama of a Buddhist temple in China, located in the outskirts of Nanjing on the road to Suzhou, I had the pleasant opportunity to be invited to visit. We went down to a cave dug into the rock where, after passing through many padlocked and chained doors, we arrived at an underground library that had survived many wars and internal revolutions in China. I was shown a collection of papyruses in rolls and some others in bamboo leaves. There was one written entirely with a monk's blood that he extracted and used as ink.

I saw another that was very well protected inside a glass box. Its age was such that no one could decipher the writing, not even monks from India who specialized in very ancient scriptures. This just reinforces that speaking about origins is not possible because sources have been lost in time.

At this spiritual level, Qigong, as well as raja-yoga, allow people that practice in order to perceive "the whole" (i.e., the full interconnection of all things on this planet, whether alive or not). In deep Qigong meditation, equivalent to the state of *samiama* in higher Yoga, the observed blends into the observer. In that state, the apparent physical separation between objects and animals disappears, and we realize that we are all part of something bigger and that separation is only an illusion. Due to these experiences or events, this type of Qigong is classified as something different or superior (also called spiritual). It is at this level that one may perceive what the ancients called "revelations." Or, in plainer terms, it's like unveiling a mystery, removing the veil of darkness and ignorance that covered it).

These achievements are similar to what the ancient Chinese knew as an *approach to the Tao*, which was the source of guidance for all processes in the universe beyond what exists or does not exist and prior to space and time. The Tao is the principle that imposes order after the ceaseless flow of change, being the origin of everything. Because of this, it is also the constant that encompasses all aspects of reality, so in this sense it can be compared to the concept of wholeness in Western philosophy (although the East says that we in the West have personified this concept with our representations of God).

My best wishes of success for the people who will try to make it to these higher states, but they should be reminded that it is usually a side effect, since the very attempt to achieve them, which is a desire, hinders its achievement.

CHAPTER 19

Recommendations and Suggestions

A good start is paramount for any human activity. It is like choosing a road from among several alternatives to reach a destination. Only if we take the right route will we reach our destination quickly and smoothly.

Simply buying a book or a video of Qigong exercises, studying the images and poses, and then imitating or replicating those described positions and exercises would be of no value; it could even be counterproductive. We should avoid the misconception that Qigong is another fitness method. It is very important to have the guidance of an experienced guide or master at the beginning in order to take advantage of the transmitted knowledge so as to not make mistakes that in some cases could produce irreversible harm. In our daily lives we often make use of guides and instructors—like the instructor who teaches us to drive a vehicle, the gym coach that shows us how to warm up our muscles before exercising, the person who teaches us to cook or play an instrument, and so on. Likewise learning Qigong requires a guide, especially since the practice involves working with energies that are very risky. We wouldn't let a person work on electrical wires without technical knowledge, for this could lead to injury or even produce a fatal shock. So it is with Qigong.

A number of positions are described in some variants of Qigong, much like the asanas[141] in yoga. These should not be seen only as a series of movements and positions to be memorized. What matters is not the movements or positions as such. We said earlier that the success of Qigong and similar activities (Reiki and Yoga) involves the body-mind interaction in one activity, and this is especially true for Qigong, where these exercises should be performed during an altered state as has been defined before. The wrongly practiced Qigong can produce damage that is not immediately apparent but appears after some time as joint damage and malfunctioning of internal secretion glands.

The benefits of the practice of Qigong are slow to manifest. We should not expect miracles immediately after only a few minutes of practice. It is clear that when a master applies Qigong as curative therapy or when acting in self-defense, its effects are immediate and almost miraculous, but to achieve this capability and level, much time and effort are required.

When you start learning and training in Qigong, whatever school, keep in mind that you should follow several stages in strict sequence:

1. **Understand** the scientific principles that underpin it.
2. **Perceive** energy and its effects on the body.
3. **Internalize** and learn about energy **accumulation and preservation.**
4. Learn to **circulate** energy internally.
5. And in the case of healing Qigong, learn to **irradiate**, **conduct,** and **apply** power qi.

Similarly, as a reference it is worth remembering a few simple rules transmitted by masters based on their long experience. These rules

---

141 Asana is a term for various postures useful for restoring and maintaining a yoga practitioner's well-being and improving the body's flexibility and vitality, with the goal of cultivating the ability to remain in seated meditation for extended periods. Asanas are widely known as "yoga postures" or "yoga positions." *Asana* quite simply means "a posture." Any way that we may sit, stand, or position our hands is an asana. And so, many asanas are possible.

comprise three basic aspects of practicing Qigong—where, when, and how—that is, the place, the time, and the manner.

Where

In general Qigong practices are focused on the individual practitioner, but it can be conducted as a group activity, especially in the learning phase. But primarily you have to remember that it is very private and individual since mind-body interaction cannot be shared. Although there might be other practicing people around, each of them would be in a kind of separate world. It is not recommended in the presence of pets (birds, cats, dogs) or close to very young children (infants). The ideal place to practice is in a quiet location, not subject to interruptions. There should not be any drafts or extreme temperatures, nor should you practice in rain, snow, or under a hot sun.

When

Most of us are subject to many pressures and commitments, so the time we can devote to this activity is strongly affected by many factors. Choosing a practice site also involves choosing a certain time, as a place that is quiet at certain hours could be different later on with the presence of a lot of people. That would be the case of a public park that very early is nearly deserted but later on starts to fill with people. For the monks who practiced Qigong in the monasteries, place and time were easy to coordinate.

The advice from the masters is to practice at sunrise or at sunset or at both times. It is not good to practice before bedtime because circadian sleep cycles are disrupted. Practice is not recommended immediately after completing any hard physical exercise or after having sex. There must be a period of rest before practicing Qigong.

Women are not recommended to practice during their menstrual periods, as it can increase blood flow and in extreme cases cause bleeding. In the event of any illness, one should consult his or her guide, master, or doctor before practicing Qigong, although in many cases it may be advisable because it accelerates the healing process and increases the defenses and immunity. In some cases, however, it might be counterproductive because it may encourage or accelerate a disease, causing bleeding or increasing degenerative processes. For this last reason, it is not recommended to apply healing Qigong in patients with terminal illnesses.

How

The way to practice Qigong comprises two phases preparation and implementation.

Regarding preparation, it should be taken into account (as explained before) that the practice requires a tight mind-body relationship, and therefore the mind must be free of heavy stress, especially in the early stages in which the practitioner has not acquired skills to reduce the distance between mind and body. Concern about diseases and daily household or work problems—either our own or those of close relatives—cause us stress. Stress seems to be constantly hammering our minds, but once you are able to acquire some skill in Qigong practices, they will in turn ease tensions caused by life's problems. At the beginning the practitioner frequently cannot achieve a good session of Qigong because his mind is disturbed. He may be worried about time commitments—getting out before a specific time to avoid traffic or arrive in time to catch a flight, attend a meeting, or keep an appointment. The beginner in these cases will be more focused on the appointment than the practice. Thus it's healthier to resolve commitments first and proceed to practice only when relaxed.

Something very important is to avoid conditionings or habituations; practicing novices run the risk of becoming dependent on them. Therefore it is not recommended to use any music during practice. It is advisable as well to avoid chemicals such as incense or aromatic candles.

Finally it is worth remembering that bodily poses in the recommended exercises were chosen based on experience. Generally those selected allow optimal relaxation of the muscles with continued normal breathing in order to not hinder mental concentration (to gain access to the altered states of consciousness).

After all this analysis and commentary, it is up to the reader to initiate in this millenary practice. Please receive my best wishes. It will be rewarding, satisfying, and full of surprises.

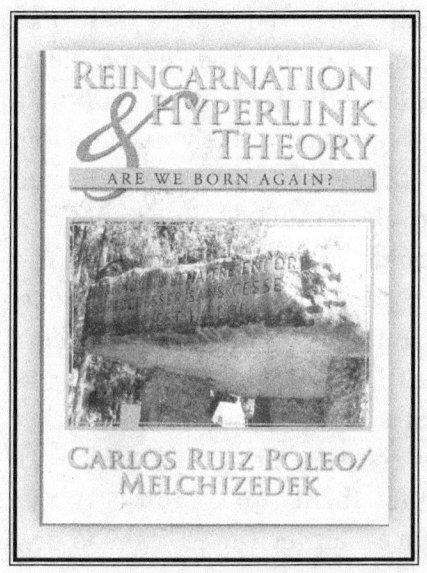

ISBN13 Hardcover: 978-1-4797-8827-9
ISBN13 Softcover: 978-1-4797-8826-2
ISBN13 e-Book: 978-1-4797-8828-6
Order online at www.xlibris.com
www.amazon.com or
www.barnesandnoble.com

A vision of someone so far unknown to him and a series of personal experiences shatter the religious convictions of the author as he struggles for more than twenty years to find a logical explanation for several interconnected events and premonitory dreams. In the search for his possible connection with the man in the dream, probably an ex-president of the United States, he analyzes several theories. But he blatantly refuses to accept past-life memories as his own because there is no scientific approach to justify their presence in his mind. There was no previous brain input or physical recording process, and no input means no memories.

As a result, a theory forms in the author's mind—reincarnation hyperlink theory—that could offer a rational explanation for the access to memories corresponding to past lives. Based on his theory, now it is easier to justify and accept the existence of past lives.

www.ruizpoleo.com

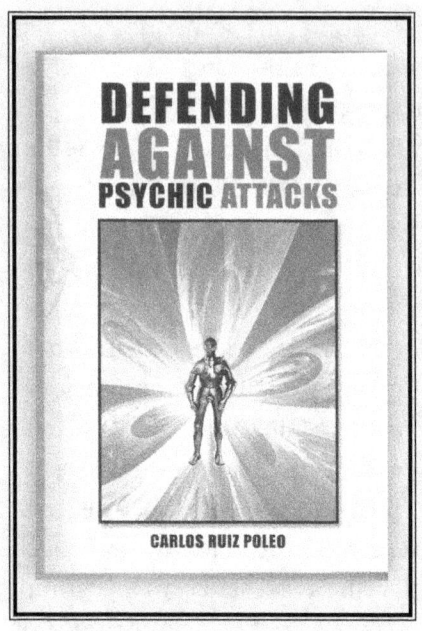

ISBN13 Hardcover: 978-1-4836-4748-7
ISBN13 Softcover: 978-1-4836-4747-0
ISBN13 e-Book: 978-1-4836-4749-4

Many of us have had bad experiences or unexpected problems in our daily lives, problems without a logical cause or a likely explanation. Some things do not go as expected despite all our efforts, and sometimes we are victims of unforeseen accidents.

We do not know why these events occur, but most people attribute them to "bad luck" or something that was "meant to be." Other people, either by superstition or rightly sustained, attribute them to a third party's influence—an "evil-eyed" person or a "bird of ill omen." And some attribute causes to premeditated attacks from witches or sorcerers who make them the target of curses or spells.

Negative intentions that could be either normal or enhanced are what we call psychic attacks. Their existence, though undeniable, is blindly rejected by many. Superstitions and myths are analyzed into a logical, rational, and partly scientific framework.

www.ruizpoleo.com